Ultrasound-guided Regional Blocks

Ultrasound-guided Regional Blocks

Pooja Gurnal
MD (Anesthesia)
Assistant Professor
Department of Anesthesia
All India Institutes of Medical Sciences
Bilaspur, Himachal Pradesh, India

Lokesh Rana
MD (Radiology)
Associate Professor
Department of Radiology
All India Institutes of Medical Sciences
Bilaspur, Himachal Pradesh, India

JAYPEE

JAYPEE BROTHERS MEDICAL PUBLISHERS
The Health Sciences Publisher
New Delhi | London

Jaypee Brothers Medical Publishers (P) Ltd

Headquarters
EMCA House, 23/23-B
Ansari Road, Daryaganj
New Delhi 110 002, India
Landline: +91-11-23272143, +91-11-23272703
+91-11-23282021, +91-11-23245672
e-mail: jaypee@jaypeebrothers.com

Corporate Office
4838/24, Ansari Road, Daryaganj
New Delhi 110 002, India
Phone: +91-11-43574357
Fax: +91-11-43574314
e-mail: jaypee@jaypeebrothers.com

Overseas Office
JP Medical Ltd.
83, Victoria Street, London
SW1H 0HW (UK)
Phone: +44-20 3170 8910
e-mail: info@jpmedpub.com

EU GPSR Authorised Representative
Logos Europe, 9 rue Nicolas Poussin
17000, La Rochelle, France
Phone: +33 (0) 6 67 93 73 78
e-mail: contact@logoseurope.eu

Website: www.jaypeebrothers.com
Website: www.jaypeedigital.com

Inquiries for bulk sales may be solicited at: jaypee@jaypeebrothers.com

Ultrasound-guided Regional Blocks

First Edition: **2026**

ISBN: 978-93-7202-827-0

Printed at: Sterling Graphics Pvt. Ltd. India.

Preface

Ultrasound guidance has revolutionized regional anesthesia and interventional pain management by allowing real-time visualization of anatomy and needle trajectory, thereby improving both efficacy and safety. This book, *Ultrasound-guided Regional Blocks,* is written jointly by specialists in anesthesia and radiology to provide a comprehensive yet practical knowledge base for clinicians. Drawing on our own clinical practice and an extensive review of current literature, we aim to integrate technical, anatomical, and procedural perspectives into a single, evidence-based resource.

Designed for anesthetists, surgeons, interventional radiologists, and trainees in these fields, the book covers the commonly practiced nerve blocks with step-by-step approaches, high-quality ultrasound images, and concise guidance. By uniting cross-disciplinary expertise, it seeks to enhance confidence, precision, and patient safety for all who perform ultrasound-guided nerve blocks.

Pooja Gurnal
Lokesh Rana

Acknowledgments

We sincerely acknowledge Dr Narvir S Chauhan, Professor of Radiology, All India Institutes of Medical Sciences (AIIMS), Bilaspur, Himachal Pradesh, India; Dr Vijalaskhmi S, Additional Professor of Anesthesia, AIIMS, Bilaspur; Dr Varun Bansal, Assistant Professor of Radiology; the Faculty Members of the Department of Anesthesia, AIIMS, Bilaspur; the Radiology Faculty, Indira Gandhi Medical College and Hospital (IGMCH), Shimla; and the Anesthesia Faculty at IGMCH, Shimla.

We also acknowledge Dr Dileep Chowdary, Senior Resident (Radiology); Arpit Singh, Radiology Technician; and Basant Thakur, MTS, Radiology.

A very special thanks to our son, Manvendra Singh.

Acknowledgements

Contents

SECTION 1

Fundamentals of Ultrasound-guided Regional Anesthesia

CHAPTER 1

Introduction to Ultrasound-guided Regional Anesthesia

PART I: ULTRASOUND PHYSICS—BASIC PRINCIPLES

As we know, diagnostic ultrasound is an important and powerful tool which is minimally invasive that improves diagnostic and therapeutic accuracy in clinical settings of the medical field. Knowledge of the basic principles of ultrasound physics form basis of image acquisition, image optimization and image integration for minimally invasive procedures such as ultrasound-guided regional anesthesia.[1] The awareness of this knowledge of imaging manipulations and ultrasound physics role in it empowers the sonologists as well as anesthetist doing the guided procedure for optimization of their clinical use in various clinical settings.[2]

Sound is a mechanical form of energy that propagates in high- and low-pressure waves in an alternative fashion, and it requires medium which in clinical setting can be air, water, fluid, tissues, and bones. Through these media, sound waves propagate in high pressure and low-pressure phases, which are called compression and rarefaction, respectively.[1,3]

Ultrasound is high-frequency sound waves to aid in diagnosis as well as various therapeutic procedures involved in patient management, and the frequencies range from 2 to 20 MHz. The transducer is an instrument which can emit as well as receive ultrasound waves which is done with the help of the piezoelectrical crystals which convert electrical signal to sound waves and vice versa.[3] These ultrasound waves or pulses of sound emitted from the transducer are propagated through the tissues and produce echoes, which are of different strength, direction and timing from different tissues, that are returned to the transducer. These returned echoes are further converted back to electrical signals by the transducer, itself and further processing is done of these signals and image we see on ultrasound screen is formed.[4] As there is difference in density on surface of the different tissues, the reflection of the ultrasound waves will be different proportional to the difference in impedance, which means if the density of tissue is high, the amount of reflected sound will also be increased in proportion whereas its proportion being transmitted will be less.[5,6] There is no production of echoes in homogenous fluids such as blood, urine, pleural effusion, and ascites because there is no difference between the tissue densities or their interfaces. Whereas if the tissue density is different, then sound is completely reflected known as acoustic shadowing as seen in calculi, bones, air, etc.[4,7,8]

Frequency is a term used to describe the number of cycles in second emitted by the probe, and its unit is Hz (hertz).[9,10] Amplitude is the height of wave and is the distance between the peak and average of a wave, power is square of the amplitude, measure in watts or milliwatts and usually displayed on ultrasound machine as dB (decibels). Acoustic impedance is the speed of ultrasound waves in soft tissue, i.e., 1,540 m/sec and as the tissue density increases, the propagation speed increases. The angle of incidence is the angle at which the ultrasound waves engage with any structure on its way. The reflectivity is maximum when the object is visualized perpendicular to the angle of the ultrasound beam.[1,10,11]

The awareness of this knowledge of ultrasound physics and its role in image manipulation make the sonologists as well as anesthetists do the guided procedure to optimize it for clinical use in various clinical settings.

PART II: THE ULTRASOUND EQUIPMENT AND KNOBOLOGY

The technological advances lead to dramatic evolvement of use of ultrasonography; however, the basic principles and functions remain essentially same.[12] For optimal performance of ultrasound-guided regional anesthesia, the knowledge as well as awareness of ultrasound knobs and equipment is important. The knowledge of the management of images generated through these knobs help us to become familiar with knobs as well as machine and optimize the ultrasound-guided procedures.[13]

ULTRASOUND PROBE OR TRANSDUCER[12,14]

These can be labeled as true workhorses of ultrasonography equipment that is an instrument, which can emit as well as receive ultrasound waves, which is done with the help of the piezoelectrical crystals, which convert electrical signals to sound waves and vice versa and generate images from returned echoes from tissues. The commonly used probes are:

- *Linear array:* High frequency (5–15 MHz) and is ideal for superficial soft tissue evaluation, neurovascular structures thus standing apart as the true workhorse for ultrasonography-guided regional anesthesia.
- *Curved array:* Low frequency (2–5 MHz) with large footprint referred as abdominal probe
- *Endocavitary:* Moderate frequency (8–15 MHz) and ideal for transvaginal use
- *Hockey stick:* High frequency (6–20 MHz) and ideal for musculoskeletal imaging and interventions

Modes

- B-mode (brightness mode) is a standard scanning mode that creates a 2-dimensional grayscale image on the ultrasound screen.[12,13]
- M-mode (motion mode) gives motion versus time display which detects motion/dynamic change in a specific location on image over a period of time.[13]
- Color Doppler mode makes use of Doppler shift, i.e., an evoked change in frequency of the returning movement to determine movement red implies that flow is toward the ultrasound probe and blue means that the flow is away from the ultrasound probe.[14,15]
- *Power Doppler mode:* It is also color Doppler but without assigning color to direction but uses shades of color commonly yellow; this mode is useful in low flow conditions.[12-15]
- Spectral Doppler allows assessment and quantification of flow velocity at specific point on an image.[15,16]

Presets: Numerous presets are available on machines which labeled as MSK, cardiac, abdominal, etc., thus, equivalent to automatically selecting particular frequency, depth and gain ideal for particular scan one needs to perform.

Power button: Mixture of "0" which indicates off and "1" which indicates on, thus a binary numbering system.

Depth: This determines how deep one wants the ultrasound machine to scan.

Gain: This makes the image brighter or darker.

Time gain compensation: This tailors the gain in near or far field as per requirement.

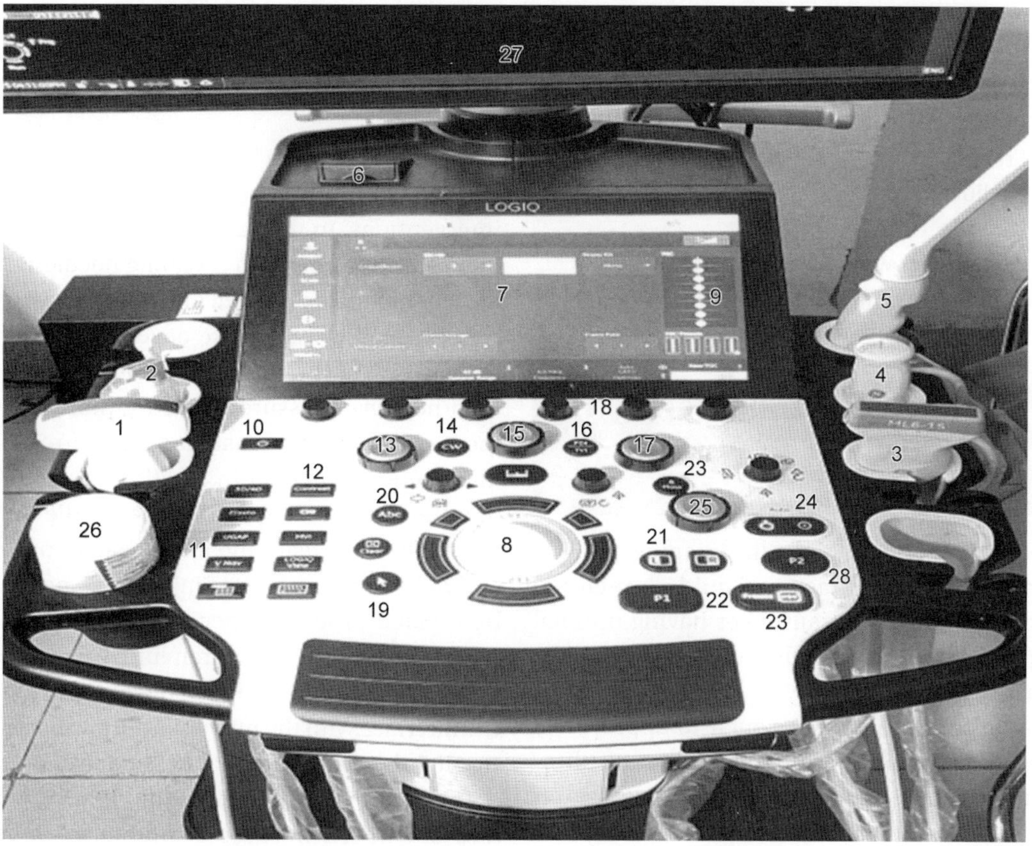

Fig. 1: Knobology of the ultrasound machine marked 1–28.

Focus: Adjusting the focus at specific depth leads to concentration of ultrasound waves, thus maximizing the resolution of the image.

Freeze: It freezes the particular desire frame thus more detailed evaluation can be done.

Caliper: It is an important knob, which enables the user to measure specific region of interest.[15-18]

Optimal performance of ultrasound-guided regional anesthesia requires proper understanding of machine, equipment and knobs **(Fig. 1)**.

Knobology:

1. Curved array transducer
2. Hockey stick transducer
3. Linear array transducer
4. Phased array transducer
5. Endo cavitary transducer
6. USB port
7. Touch screen panel
8. Track ball
9. Time gain compensation
10. Power button
11. Advanced application presets
12. Advanced image improvement features
13. M-mode
14. Continuous wave Doppler
15. Pulsed wave Doppler
16. Power Doppler imaging
17. Color flow
18. Soft keys to adjust options on touch screen

19. Pointer options
20. Annotations
21. Splitting screen or dual screen option
22. Print and save buttons
23. Freeze
24. Audio options
25. B-mode
26. Gel warmer with ultrasound gel bottle
27. USG display monitor
28. Saving button for cine clips and videos

PART III: NEEDLE VISUALIZATION AND GUIDANCE TECHNIQUES AND TRICKS

The optimization of needle imaging plays a pivotal role in ultrasound-guided regional blocks. Appropriate transducer having optimal frequency needs to be selected, then one has to do assessment of anatomy.[8]

Adjusting the patient couch to appropriate height and ergonomically placement of ultrasound machine is important as it gives better hand eye movements on the patient as well as screen.[8,19,20]

Pressure is applied on the transducer in a variable amount in real time visualizing sonographic anatomy, alignment with underlying nerve is done, fine tuning if required done with rotation and tilting of the probe with optimal anatomic recognition of the target nerve.[8,20-22]

Nerve imaging may be done along short axis where the probe is perpendicular to nerve axis, or the probe is in long axis where the probe is parallel to axis of the nerve, but it is more often seen that interventionist/anesthetist having probe and needle aligned to his/her axis. Preblock scan with Doppler analysis is highly recommended to do preintervention planning.[23]

The maintenance of needle tip visualization and advancing it avoiding injury to vital structures is of utmost importance and is achieved by using a shallow angle, heeling of one end of transducer, rotating and tilting for better visualization and use of echogenic needle which are available nowadays.[24]

"Hydro-location" is the technique/trick which has proven to be beneficial in majority of interventions. In this, a small amount of fluid is injected, which helps in revealing needle tip and its path better, especially if difficult situation.[23,24]

On obtaining adequate needle placement in the vicinity of the nerve which is targeted and with negative pressure to ensure that tip is not located inside intravascular structure. Local anesthetic is injected in small doses ensuring that the injectate is spread at the needle tip and is visualized in real time and negative pressure still to be given. A halo of injectate is needed to be created around, especially solitary nerves. Another tip to prevent intraneural injection and nerve injury is that when the needle has reached the interface with the nerve, withdraw the needle tip slightly and ensure that nerve does not move along with needle tip retraction. Fascial planes and sheaths, wherever available, should be taken use of in the optimal spread of the local anesthetic injectate along the longitudinal axials of the nerve.[8,25]

REFERENCES

1. Grogan SP, Mount CA. Ultrasound physics and instrumentation. In: StatPearls. StatPearls Publishing; 2023.
2. AIUM Curriculum for Fundamentals of Ultrasound Physics and Instrumentation. J Ultrasound Med. 2019;38(8):1933-5.
3. Aldrich JE. Basic physics of ultrasound imaging. Crit Care Med. 2007;35(Suppl 5):S131-7.
4. Nadrljanski M, Murphy A, Hacking C, et al. Physical principles of ultrasound. Reference article, Radiopaedia.org (Accessed on 19 Apr 2025) https://doi.org/10.53347/rID-8663
5. Shriki J. Ultrasound physics. Crit Care Clin. 2014;30(1):1-24, v.

6. Huang J, Li J, Wang H. The Principles and Procedures of Ultrasound-guided Anesthesia Techniques. Cureus. 2018;10(7):e2980.
7. Lawrence JP. Physics and instrumentation of ultrasound. Crit Care Med. 2007;35(8 Suppl): S314-22.
8. Orebaugh SL, Kirkham KR. Introduction to ultrasound-guided regional anesthesia. Nysora; 2022.
9. Lieu D. Ultrasound physics and instrumentation for pathologists. Arch Pathol Lab Med. 2010; 134(10):1541-56.
10. Lieu D. Ultrasound fundamentals and their clinical implications for interventional cytopathologists. Cytopathology. 2025;36(4):356-74.
11. Staren ED. Physics and principles of breast ultrasound. Am Surg. 1996;62(2):103-7.
12. Bahner DP, Blickendorf JM, Bockbrader M, Adkins E, Vira A, Boulger C, et al. Language of Transducer Manipulation. J Ultrasound Med. 2016;35:183-8.
13. Enriquez JL, Wu TS. An introduction to ultrasound equipment and knobology. Crit Care Clin. 2014; 30(1):25-45.
14. Rosenberg I, Schwarzenbach HR, Tuma J. «Knopfologie» (Wichtige Geräteeinstellungen) [«Knobology» (important device settings)]. Praxis (Bern 1994). 2012;101(18):1207-12.
15. AIUM technical bulletin. Transducer manipulation. American Institute of Ultrasound in Medicine. J Ultrasound Med. 1999;18(2):169-75.
16. Balbis S, Meloni T, Tofani S, Zenone F, Nucera D, Guiot C. Criteria and scheduling of quality control of B-mode and doppler ultrasonography equipment. J Clin Ultrasound. 2012;40(3):167-73.
17. Trier HG. Funktionseigenschaften von Ultraschalldiagnostikgeräten. Ein Konzept von Prüfbausteinen zur Durchführung der Qualitätssicherung [Functional properties of diagnostic ultrasound instruments. A concept of trial building blocks for implementing quality assurance]. Ultraschall Med. 1994;15(5):223-32.
18. Vicki EN, Nelson B. Manual of Emergency and Critical Care Ultrasound. Cambridge: Cambridge UP; 2011.
19. Chin KJ, Perlas A, Chan VW, Brull R. Needle visualization in ultrasound-guided regional anesthesia: challenges and solutions. Reg Anesth Pain Med. 2008;33(6):532-44.
20. Frohlich J, Sancheti S. Hydrolocation assisted subclavian venous catheterization-two case reports. Korean J Anesthesiol. 2022;75(5): 445-8.
21. Kapral S, Krafft P, Eibenberger K, Fitzgerald R, Gosch M, Weinstabl C. Ultrasound-guided supraclavicular approach for regional anesthesia of the brachial plexus. Anesth Analg. 1994;78: 507-13.
22. Marhofer P, Schrogendofer K, Koinig H, Kapral S, Weinstabl C, Mayer N. Ultasonographic guidance improves sensory block and onset time of three-in-one blocks. Anesth Analg. 1997;85:854-7.
23. Alakkad H, Chin KJ. The importance of good needling technique in ultrasound-guided axillary block. Reg Anesth. 2013;38(2):166.
24. Tsui BC. Facilitating needle alignment in-plane to an ultrasound beam using a portable laser unit. Reg Anesth Pain Med. 2007;32:84-8.
25. Wong SW, Niazi AU, Chin KJ, Chan VW. Real-time ultrasound guided spinal anesthesia using the SonixGPS® needle tracking system. Can J Anaesth. 2013;60:50-3.

SECTION 2

Upper Limb Blocks

CHAPTER 2

Interscalene Block

INTRODUCTION

The brachial plexus is formed by C5-T1 and is a nerve network that supplies upper extremity. As it exits, the cervical spine travels between the anterior and middle scalene muscles.[1,2] The space between the scalene muscles is called interscalene groove.

The interscalene block (ISB) was first conceptualized in 1970, and it is increasingly becoming common in upper limb surgeries.[1] The ISB under ultrasound guidance has faster onset of time and longer duration compared to nerve stimulation technique, resulting in more reliable surgical anesthesia for the same volume of local anesthetic agent.[3,4] Under the ultrasound guidance, local anesthetic delivery and adequate spread around the brachial plexus can be ensured. Performing the block using the peri plexus approach, i.e., outside the brachial plexus sheath under ultrasound guidance may reduce the risk of nerve injury.[5]

IMPORTANT ANATOMICAL CONSIDERATIONS[6]

- The phrenic nerve, which runs anterolaterally to the anterior scalene muscle, may be injured causing hemiparesis of diaphragm.
- The vertebral artery lying medially whereas the internal jugular vein and carotid artery are anteromedial to the brachial plexus.
- The cervical plexus and stellate ganglion are in close proximity, influencing side effects.

INDICATIONS[7,8]

- Shoulder surgeries
- Proximal humerus fracture
- Clavicle surgeries
- Pain management for chronic shoulder pain (e.g., frozen shoulder, etc.)

CONTRAINDICATIONS[8]

- *Absolute:*
  - Local anesthetic allergy
  - Patient refusal
  - Infection at the local site
  - Lack of skilled assistance
  - Lack of resuscitation equipment
- *Relative:*
  - Deranged coagulation profile
  - Systemic infection
  - Preexisting injury of brachial plexus and its nerves distally

EQUIPMENT[3,8,9]

Healthcare professionals performing ISB should be equipped with the following items:

- Standard physiological monitors [electrocardiogram (ECG), BP apparatus, and pulse oximeter]
- Resuscitation equipment
- Ultrasound machine with a high frequency linear transducer
- Sterile gloves, drapes, and ultrasonography (USG) probe covers
- Skin antiseptics, e.g., betadine, alcohol, and chlorhexidine

- Two inch, 22-gauge, short beveled, insulated, and stimulating needle
- A 3-mL syringe with a 25-gauge needle with local anesthetic agent for skin infiltration
- One 20–30 mL syringe with local anesthetic
- Marking pen

PERSONNEL

The ISB block requires two persons, one to control the ultrasound probe and needle, another to manage the syringe and inject local anesthetic.

ULTRASOUND-GUIDED INTERSCALENE BLOCK TECHNIQUE

- Gain intravenous access, apply standard monitors, and perform standard safety check list.[10,11]
- *Patient positioning:* The patient can be positioned in supine, sitting, semi-sitting, or lateral decubitus, most commonly done with semi-sitting position with support of pillow or blanket given beneath the patient chest with head rotated toward contralateral side and the area on the neck adequately exposed. Care must be taken that the patient should be able to lie comfortably and still.[3,8]
- *Transducer positioning:* Two approaches are commonly employed for proper image structure are identified **(Figs. 1A and B)**.[3]
  - In the first method, the transducer is placed medial to sternocleidomastoid muscle at the level of cricoid cartilage, and the carotid artery is identified, then the transducer is slid laterally until between the anterior and middle scalene the brachial plexus is identified.
  - In the second method, transducer is placed just above the clavicle, and subclavian artery is identified, transducer is then moved cephalad toward patient neck with keeping the brachial plexus nerves in profile until the image with "stop light" sign is seen.[12] The C6 nerve root fascicles are correctly identified by tracing where it exits the intervertebral foramen. Color Doppler should be used to identify vascular structures with attention paid to avoid vertebral artery and the transverse cervical artery.[13,14]

BRACHIAL PLEXUS INTERSCALENE BLOCK CONDUCT[3,8,15-17]

- After confirming the critical landmarks, anterior scalene, middle scalene, and C5–C6 roots in interscalene groove skin are infiltered with 1–3 mL local anesthetic.
- The block needle is advanced in plane through skin and medial scalene toward the C5–C6 roots lying in interscalene groove.
- Advance the needle through the medial scalene and just stop at the border of its fascial layer with the hyperechoic fascia covering the brachial plexus.
- Feel the subtle "pop" sensation when the needle tip enters the interscalene groove. The peri plexus approach is adopted by not piercing the sheath of brachial plexus as there is less chance of nerve injury.
- Aspiration is done to rule out intravascular position of needle tip and then inject 1 mL of saline to confirm the needle tip position between the fascial layers.
- Inject gently with low pressure and rule out nerve expansion due to intraneural injection, do communicate with the patient ask for paresthesia during needle advancements.
- If the injectate spread posteriorly along the needle tract along medial scalene then advance 1–2 mm further avoiding intraneural injection
- The correct injection is denoted by deposition which will appear on ultrasound as the plexus pushed medially with hypoechoic spread adjacent to the nerve roots. Local anesthetics

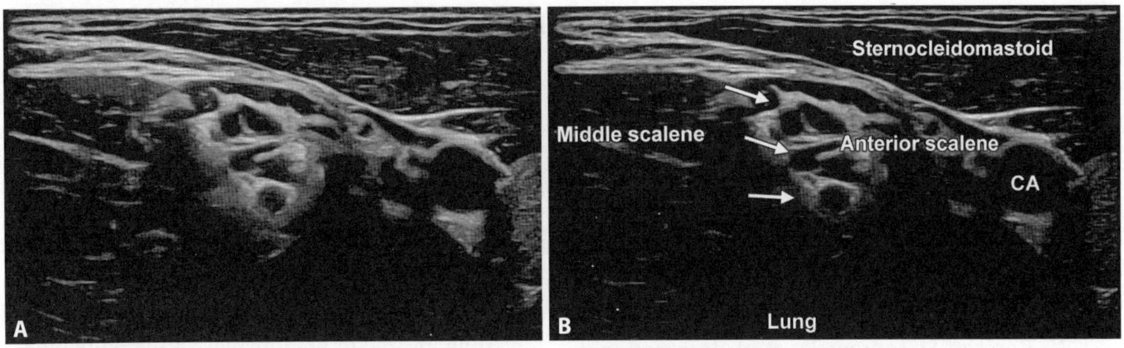

Figs. 1A and B: Sonographic anatomy from superficial to deep plane showing brachial plexus (arrows) seen between the anterior and middle scalene muscle at the supraclavicular fossa below the cricoid cartilage and medial to sternocleidomastoid muscle and carotid artery (CA).

must visualize within the correct tissue plane in the interscalene groove, and complete circumferential spread around the plexus is not necessary.

- Once satisfactory needle position is obtained, inject desired local anesthetic volume in small 3–5 mL increments in low pressure aspirating intermittently to rule out intravascular injection. The overall local anesthetic dose should be <2.5 mg/kg with usual dose of 15–30 mL of 0.25 bupivacaine or 0.2% ropivacaine.

SIDE EFFECTS[8,15]

- Horner's syndrome
- Phrenic nerve block
- Recurrent laryngeal nerve block

COMPLICATIONS[3]

- Infection
- Bleeding/hematoma
- Local anesthetic toxicity
- Intravascular toxicity
- Epidural or subarachnoid injection
- Pneumothorax
- Permanent nerve injury
- Injury to long or dorsal scapular nerves
- Injury to brachial plexus nerve roots

SUMMARY

- The ISB is given to provide analgesia and anesthesia to the shoulder and proximal arm by blocking C5–6 nerve roots.
- Linear high frequency transducer is used to identify the nerve roots in the interscalene groove done by tracing the brachial plexus proximal from the supraclavicular level.
- The needle tip is positioned in the potential space between the medial scalene and the brachial plexus sheath with use of a peri plexus approach of safe and effective local anesthetic deposition.
- The common complications and side effects include injury to the brachial plexus, pneumothorax, diaphragmatic palsy, and recurrent laryngeal nerve palsy.

REFERENCES

1. Takayama K, Shiode H, Ito H. Ultrasound-guided interscalene block anesthesia performed by an orthopedic surgeon: a study of 1322 cases of shoulder surgery. JSES Int. 2022;6(1):149-54.
2. Kapral S, Greher M, Huber G, Willschke H, Kettner S, Kdolsky R, et al. Ultrasonographic guidance improves the success rate of interscalene brachial plexus blockade. Reg Anesth Pain Med. 2008;33(3):253-8.

3. Zisquit J, Nedeff N. Interscalene Block. In: StatPearls. StatPearls Publishing, Treasure Island (FL); 2025. PMID: 30137775.
4. Xu D. Hadzic's Peripheral Nerve Blocks and Anatomy for Ultrasound-Guided Regional Anesthesia, 2nd edition.
5. Szerb JJ, Greenberg MJ, Kwofie MM, Baldridge WH, Zhou PR, Wong PK. Reports of original investigations. Can J Anesth/J Can Anesth. 2015;62:1295-302.
6. Bowness JS, Pawa A, Turbitt L, Bellew B, Bedforth N, Burckett-St Laurent D, et al. International consensus on anatomical structures to identify on ultrasound for the performance of basic blocks in ultrasound-guided regional anesthesia. Reg Anesth Pain Med. 2022;47(2):106-12.
7. Pester JM, Hendrix JM, Hendrix JM, Varacallo MA. Brachial Plexus Block Techniques. In: StatPearls. StatPearls Publishing, Treasure Island (FL); 2025. PMID: 29262036
8. Vierula M, Robert J, Wong P, McVicar J. Ultrasound-Guided Interscalene Block. Reg Anesth. WFSA; 2019.
9. Hanson NA, Auyong DB. Systematic ultrasound identification of the dorsal scapular and long thoracic nerves during interscalene block. Reg Anesth Pain Med. 2013;38(1):54-7.
10. Mulroy MF, Weller RS, Liguori GA. A checklist for performing regional nerve blocks. Reg Anesth Pain Med. 2014;39(3):195-9.
11. Gul F, Nazir M, Abbas K, Khan AA, Malick DS, Khan H, et al. Surgical safety checklist compliance: The clinical audit. Ann Med Surg. 2022;81:104397.
12. Franco CD, Williams JM. Ultrasound-guided interscalene block: reevaluation of the "stoplight" sign and clinical implications. Reg Anesth Pain Med. 2016;41(4):452-9.
13. van Geffen GJ, Moayeri N, Bruhn J, Scheffer GJ, Chan VW, Groen GJ. Correlation between ultrasound imaging, cross-sectional anatomy, and histology of the brachial plexus: a review. Reg Anesth Pain Med. 2009;34(5):490-7.
14. Martinoli C, Bianchi S, Santacroce E, Pugliese F, Graif M, Derchi LE. Brachial plexus sonography: a technique for assessing the root level. Am J Roentgenol. 2002;179(3):699-702.
15. Stasiowski M, Zuber M, Marciniak R, Kolny M, Chabierska E, Jałowiecki P, et al. Risk factors for the development of Horner's syndrome following interscalene brachial plexus block using ropivacaine for shoulder arthroscopy: a randomised trial. Anaesthesiol Intensive Ther. 2018;50(3):215-20.
16. Vester-Andersex T, Christiansen C, Hansen A, Sørensen M, Meisler C. Interscalene brachial plexus block: area of analgesia, complications and blood concentrations of local anesthetics. Acta Anaesthesiol Scand. 1981;25(2):81-4.
17. Mariano ER, Afra R, Loland VJ, Sandhu NS, Bellars RH, Bishop ML, et al. Continuous Interscalene Brachial Plexus Block via an Ultrasound-Guided Posterior Approach: A Randomized, Triple-Masked, Placebo-Controlled Study. Anesth Analg. 2009;108(5):1688-94.

CHAPTER 3

Supraclavicular Block

INTRODUCTION

The supraclavicular approach to the brachial plexus block was first introduced in 1911 by Kulenkampff, and it is arguably the most preferred with highest success rate.[1] The ultrasound guidance enables a real time visualization of the needle, and vascular and pleural structures can be identified and avoided.[2,3]

IMPORTANT ANATOMICAL CONSIDERATIONS

As the trunks/divisions of the brachial plexus with this approach are superficial to the skin, its visualization by ultrasonography (USG) is easy. It is an ideal site to achieve anesthesia due to limited surface area as plexus remains tightly packed here, so rapid and high-quality anesthesia is possible, therefore often called as "spinal of the arm".[2,3]

The supraclavicular approach targets the divisions level with block extending in the brachial plexus from the distal trunks to proximal cords.[3]

INDICATIONS[2,4,5]

- Fractures, dislocations, abscess drainage, or general surgery of upper extremity
- Analgesia (postsurgical, post-traumatic, complex pain syndrome, postamputation, and vascular and tumor-related pain)

CONTRAINDICATIONS[6,7]

- *Absolute:*
  - Local anesthetic allergy
  - Patient refusal
  - Infection at the local site
  - Lack of skilled assistance
  - Lack of resuscitation equipment
- *Relative:*
  - Deranged coagulation profile, a more superficial block to be considered as per American Society for Regional Anesthesia and Pain (ASRA)
  - Systemic infection
  - Preexisting neural deficit in the distribution of the block

EQUIPMENT[6,8,9]

Healthcare professional performing supraclavicular block should be equipped with following items:

- Standard physiological monitors [electrocardiogram (ECG), BP appratus and pulse oximeter]
- Resuscitation equipment
- Ultrasound machine with a high frequency linear transducer (10–15 MHz)
- Sterile gloves, drapes, and USG probe covers
- Skin antiseptics, e.g., betadine, alcohol, and chlorhexidine
- Local anesthetic, i.e., 2% lidociane
- Mild sedative agents, i.e., 1–2 mg of midazolam
- Regional block local anesthesia (0.5% bupivacaine/ropivacaine for postoperative analgesia and 2% lidocaine for short onset time requirement)
- Short bevel insulated, stimulating block needle 10 cm (22 gauge for single injection and

18 gauge for continuous catheter), insulated, and stimulating needle
- A 3-mL syringe with a 25-gauge needle with local anesthetic agent for skin infiltration
- One 10–20 mL syringe with local anesthetic
- Marking pen

PERSONNEL

The interscalene block requires two persons, one to control the ultrasound probe and needle, other to manage the syringe and inject local anesthetic.

ULTRASONOGRAPHY-GUIDED SUPRACLAVICULAR TECHNIQUE

- The provider must perform the process of informed consent.[6]
- Gain intravenous access, apply standard monitors and perform standard safety check list.[10]
- *Patient positioning:* The patient can be positioned in supine position with arms by the side with support of pillow or blanket given beneath the patient shoulder to improve the access to supraclavicular space also the head rotated toward contralateral side and the area on the neck adequately exposed. Care must be taken, it should be ensured that the patient is comfortable and still.
- Mild sedation with 1–2 mg of midazolam may be provided though many patients do not need it.[3,10]
- Skin antiseptics are applied to the skin, then sterile conduction gel is applied to the ultrasound transducer, and use of sterile probe cover is recommended.[3]
- *Transducer positioning and technique:* After palpation of clavicle and clavicular head of sternoclavicular muscle, the linear ultrasound transducer is placed in the supraclavicular fossa in the mid-clavicle superior aspect. The probe should be placed in a parasagittal or coronal plane with optimization done by rotating the probe for obtaining a view that contains subclavian artery, first rib, and pleura and brachial plexus trunks/divisions **(Figs. 1A and B)**.[11]
  - *First rib*: Hyperechoic bottom of the screen seen as white horizontal/oblique line, inferior to it is lung seen as gray area referred to as danger area, needle advancement below the level of first rib carries a risk of penetrating into parietal pleura resulting in pneumothorax.[12,13]

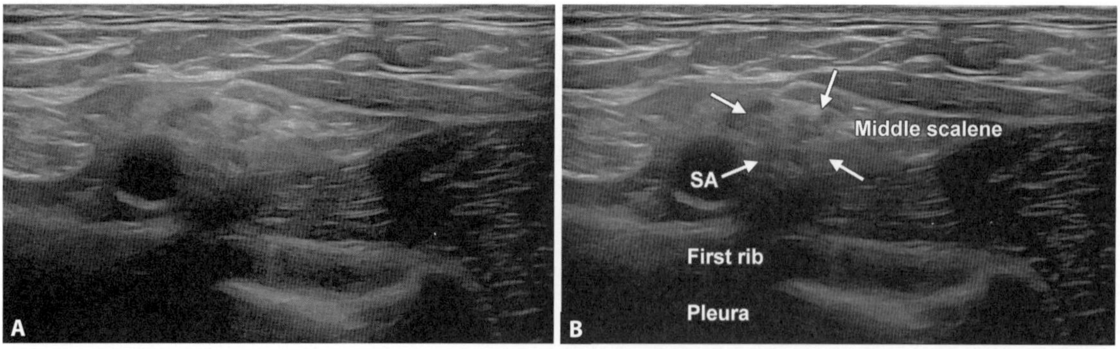

Figs. 1A and B: Supraclavicular sonographic anatomy from superficial to deep plane shows brachial plexus, which is enveloped in connective tissue seen posterolateral to subclavian artery (SA), whereas first rib and pleura are also seen in close vicinity.

- *Subclavian artery*: Pulsating, round, hypoechoic, and confirmed on color Doppler
- *Brachial plexus*: It is cephalad to subclavian artery (SCA) and seen as grape-like structures.

- After locally anesthetizing the skin with 1% lidocaine, the short-beveled needle is inserted using in-plane technique from the lateral border of the probe and the needle is advanced from the lateral to the medial direction in same plane and the entire length of needle is visualized as its tip heads toward the brachial plexus. The "corner pocket" is the ideal injection site, and it is the junction of the brachial plexus and posterolateral border of subclavian artery in the superior aspect of first rib.[14]
- On confirmation of needle tip location, the local anesthetic agent is injected between the divisions of the brachial plexus using hydro dissection technique which "floats" the plexus superficially.[13] Then, the needle is redirected toward superficial aspect of the plexus or middle of the cluster and local anesthetic injected there too.
  - For surgical procedures 20 mL of 0.5% bupivacaine
  - For analgesic block 20 mL of 0.25% bupivacaine
- The exact volume can be judged by eye balling and injection stopped once all the nerve structure has been bathed in local anesthetic solution.

SIDE EFFECTS[3,6,15]

- Horner's syndrome
- Phrenic nerve block
- Ipsilateral laryngeal nerve block

COMPLICATIONS[3,16,17]

- Infection
- Bleeding/hematoma
- Local anesthetic toxicity
- Intravascular toxicity
- Pneumothorax
- Permanent nerve injury
- Injury to brachial plexus nerve roots

SUMMARY

- The supraclavicular approach targets the distal trunks and proximal division level of brachial plexus and results in anesthesia of the upper arm distal to the shoulder.
- The improved safety is accorded by ultrasound guidance allowing the visualization of the pleura.
- The "corner pocket" is the ideal injection site and is the junction of the brachial plexus and posterolateral border of subclavian artery in the superior aspect of first rib.
- The local anesthetic agent is injected between the divisions of the brachial plexus using hydrodissection technique which "floats" the plexus superficially.

REFERENCES

1. Bharti N, Bhardawaj N, Wig J. Comparison of ultrasound-guided supraclavicular, infraclavicular and below-C6 interscalene brachial plexus block for upper limb surgery: a randomised, observer-blinded study. Anaesth Intensive Care. 2015;43(4):468-72.
2. Govender S, Möhr D, Tshabalala ZN, van Schoor A. A review of the anatomy and a step-by-step visual guide to performing an ultrasound-guided supraclavicular brachial plexus block. Southern African J Anaesth Analg. 2019;1-6.
3. Kusre S, McEwen A, Matthew G. Ultrasound-Guided Supraclavicular Brachial Plexus Block. Reg Anaesth. 2018;87(6):883.
4. Wankhade H, Chauhan VP, Parikh R, Saxena AK. Ultrasound-guided supraclavicular brachial plexus block for the upper limb fracture or dislocation reduction in emergency in emergency department. IRPMS. 2017;2(5):16-21.

5. Möhr D. When will the sonar ping reach our shores. SA J Anaesth Analg. 2010;16(3):4.
6. Ryan DJ, Iofin N, Furgiuele D, Johnson J, Egol K. Regional anesthesia for clavicle fracture surgery is safe and effective. J Shoulder Elbow Surg. 2021;30(7):e356-60.
7. Kapral S, Krafft P, Eibenberger K, Fitzgerald R, Gosch M, Weinstabl C. Ultrasound-guided supraclavicular approach for regional anesthesia of the brachial plexus. Anesth Analg. 1994;78(3):507-13.
8. Neal JM, Gerancher JC, Hebl JR, Ilfeld BM, McCartney CJ, Franco CD, et al. Upper extremity regional anesthesia: essentials of our current understanding, 2008. Reg Anesth Pain Med. 2009;34(2):134-70. [Erratum in: Reg Anesth Pain Med. 2010;35(4):407.]
9. Soares LG, Brull R, Lai J, Chan VW. Eight ball, corner pocket: the optimal needle position for ultrasound-guided supraclavicular block. Reg Anesth Pain Med. 2007;32(1):94-5.
10. Gamo K, Kuriyama K, Higuchi H, Uesugi A, Nakase T, Hamada M, et al. Ultrasound-guided supraclavicular brachial plexus block in upper limb surgery: outcomes and patient satisfaction. Bone Joint J. 2014;96-B(6):795-9.
11. Tran DQ, Munoz L, Zaouter C, Russo G, Finlayson RJ. A prospective, randomized comparison between single- and double-injection, ultrasound-guided supraclavicular brachial plexus block. Reg Anesth Pain Med. 2009;34(5):420-4.
12. Abell DJ, Barrington MJ. Pneumothorax after ultrasound-guided supraclavicular block: presenting features, risk, and related training. Reg Anesth Pain Med. 2014;39(2):164-7.
13. Demondion X, Herbinet P, Boutry N, Fontaine C, Francke JP, Cotten A. Sonographic mapping of the normal brachial plexus. Am J Neuroradiol. 2003;24(7):1303-9.
14. Christie LE, Picard J, Weiberg GL. Local anaesthetic systemic toxicity. BJA Education. 2015;15(3):136-42.
15. Association of Anaesthetists of Great Britain and Ireland. Management of severe local anaesthetic toxicity. AAGBI Safety Guideline; 2010.
16. Brown DL, Cahill DR, Bridenbaugh LD. Supraclavicular nerve block: anatomic analysis of a method to prevent pneumothorax. Anesth Analg. 1993;76(3):530-4.
17. Cave G, Harrop-Griffiths W, Harvey M, Meek T, Picard J, Short T, et al. Management of severe local anaesthetic toxicity. 2010.

CHAPTER 4

Infraclavicular Block

INTRODUCTION

The approaches to brachial plexus blocks have evolved over the time in history from landmark guidance, nerve stimulator guidance to ultrasound guidance.[1] The infraclavicular brachial plexus block, a regional anesthetic technique developed as the pneumothorax, was an occasional occurrence with supraclavicular block, though the risk is very minimal.[1,2]

IMPORTANT ANATOMICAL CONSIDERATIONS

In the brachial plexus the ventral rami of C5-T1 nerve roots which exits the intervertebral foramina and form superior, middle and inferior trunks which travels between the anterior and middle scalene muscles.[3] These three trunks branch into six divisions behind the clavicle, which join into lateral, posterior, and medial cords under the clavicle and are named as per their relative position to the axillary artery, and then cords split into five terminal branches of the brachial plexus.[4] The infraclavicular block is carried out below the clavicle at the midpoint of the cord level of the brachial plexus.[3-5] The cord is lying posterior, lateral, and medial to axillary artery, and the boundaries on sonography are anteriorly pectoralis major and minor muscles, medially ribs, superiorly clavicle and coracoid process, and humerus is laterally.[4]

INDICATIONS[3,4,6]

- Surgery of elbow, forearm, wrist, and hand
- Postoperative pain control for upper extremity surgeries
- Complex regional pain syndrome of upper extremity
- Procedures requiring anesthesia and analgesia below the mid-humerus.

CONTRAINDICATIONS[6,7]

- *Absolute:*
    - Local anesthetic allergy
    - Patient refusal
    - Infection at the local site
    - Lack of skilled assistance
    - Lack of resuscitation equipment
- *Relative:*
    - Deranged coagulation
    - Systemic infection
    - Short neck
    - Thick pectoral region
    - Dislocation or fracture of the clavicle

EQUIPMENT[4,6,8,9]

A healthcare professional performing an infraclavicular block should be equipped with the following items:

- Standard physiological monitors [electrocardiogram (ECG), BP apparatus, and pulse oximeter]
- Resuscitation equipment
- Ultrasound machine with a high-frequency linear transducer (8–15 MHz)
- Sterile gloves, drapes, and ultrasonography (USG) probe covers
- Skin antiseptics, e.g., betadine, alcohol, and chlorhexidine
- Local anesthetic, i.e., 2% lidociane

- Mild sedative agents, i.e., 1–2 mg of midazolam
- Regional block local anesthesia (0.5% bupivacaine/ropivacaine for postoperative analgesia and 2% lidocaine for short onset time requirement)
- Short bevel insulated, stimulating block needle 10 cm (22-gauge for single injection and 18-gauge for continuous catheter), insulated, stimulating needle
- A 3-mL syringe with a 25-gauge needle with a local anesthetic agent for skin infiltration
- One 10–20 mL syringe with local anesthetic
- Marking pen

PERSONNEL

The infraclavicular block requires two persons, one to control the ultrasound probe and needle and the other to manage the nerve stimulator (optional) and the syringe with local anesthetic. An additional person will monitor the vitals of the patient and will administer the emergency drugs if needed.[3,4,6]

ULTRASOUND-GUIDED INFRACLAVICULAR BLOCK TECHNIQUE

- The provider must perform the process of informed consent.[3,6]
- Gain intravenous access, apply standard monitors, and perform standard safety checklist.[3]
- *Patient positioning:* The patient can be positioned in the supine position with arms abducted and flexed at the elbow to have an optimal relationship of landmarks to the brachial plexus.[4] The head is rotated toward the contralateral side and the area on the neck adequately exposed. Care must be taken that the patient should be able to lie comfortably and still.[9]
- Mild sedation with 1–2 mg of midazolam may be provided, though many patients do not need it.[4,6,9]
- Skin antiseptic is applied to the skin, then sterile conduction gel is applied to the ultrasound transducer, and use of sterile probe cover is recommended.[6,10]
- *Transducer positioning and technique:* The pivotal structure to visualize while performing the USG-guided infraclavicular block of brachial plexus is and axillary artery, which lies in the posterior aspect of pectoralis major and minor muscles and is seen as dark, round, pulsating structure with hyperechoic walls, axillary vein lying beside the artery which is compressible and collapsible, the confirmation can be made on color Doppler **(Figs. 1A and B)**.[3,11-13] One should keep in mind that the location of the brachial plexus in the infraclavicular region is deeper, i.e., ≥4 cm, and the anatomical relation around the axillary artery can vary significantly. The three most common approaches for needle insertion are:
  1. *Vertical approach:* It is the simplest, reliable, and safest approach, so it is most commonly used. The needle is inserted anteroposteriorly immediately caudal to the middle of the clavicle at the midpoint of the infraclavicular line between the acromion and jugular fossa under ultrasound guidance for identifying the vital structure.[14]
  2. *Coracoid Approach:* The coracoid process is identified by palpation of a bony prominence, which is medial to the shoulder; the medial clavicular head is located, a line joining the two landmarks is drawn, and the midpoint is marked. The needle is inserted 2 cm medial and 2 cm inferior to the coracoid process and directed ventral to dorsal under ultrasound guidance with the cord identified at an average depth of 4.5 cm.[3,6,14,15]
  3. *Parasagittal approach:* The needle is inserted inferior to the clavicle in the

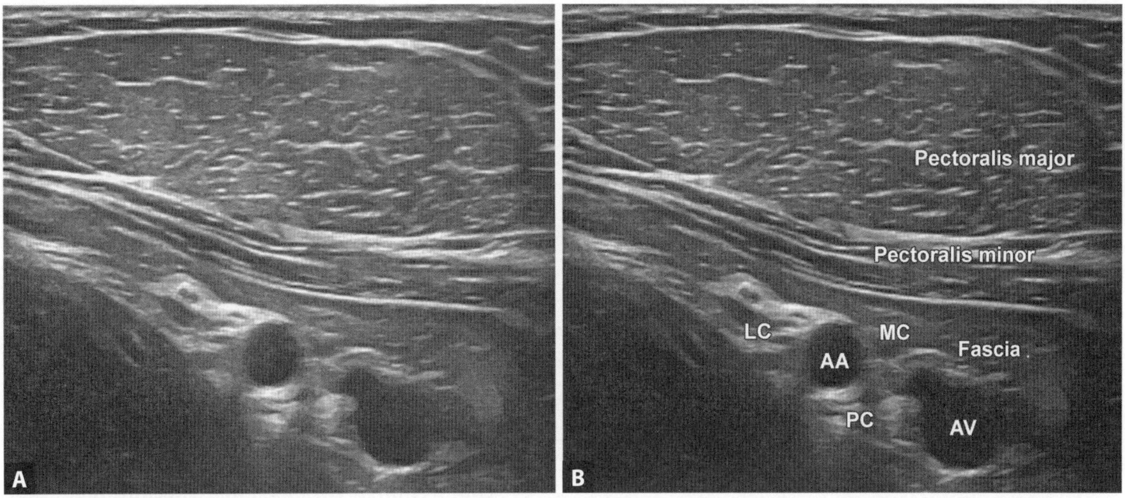

Figs. 1A and B: Sonographic anatomy of brachial plexus in the infraclavicular region from superficial to deep and labeled anatomical structures. The medial cord (MC), the posterior cord (PC), and the lateral cord (LC) are located below the fascia and around the axillary artery (AA) and axillary vein (AV).

groove between the coracoid and the clavicle under ultrasound guidance with identification of axillary artery as described above in the cephalad to caudal direction, and cords are encountered at an average distance of 5–6 cm.[16]

Other approaches have also been described as ultrasound has enabled experimental research and development of new techniques.[2,8,17]

- After locally anesthetizing the skin with 2 mL 1% lidocaine, the short-beveled block needle is inserted using an in-plane technique from cephalad to caudal direction, and the needle tip is guided as described in the approaches above. The local anesthetic is injected two-thirds of the volume posterior to the axillary artery around the posterior and medial cords, and then the needle tip is redirected by retracting toward the lateral cord, and the remaining one-third of the local anesthetic is injected. The deposit of local anesthetic in 5 mL aliquots, followed by aspiration, decreases the risk of aspiration.[4,8]
    - For surgical procedures, 20 mL of 0.5% bupivacaine
    - For an analgesic block, 20 mL of 0.25% bupivacaine
- The exact volume can be judged by eyeballing, and injection is stopped once all the nerve structure has been bathed in local anesthetic solution.

SIDE EFFECTS[11]

- Phrenic nerve block
- Pneumothorax (0.7%)
- Horner syndrome

COMPLICATIONS[18]

- Infection
- Bleeding/hematoma
- Local anesthetic toxicity
- Vascular puncture
- Intravascular toxicity
- Needle-induced paresthesia
- Permanent nerve injury
- Injury to the brachial plexus nerve roots

SUMMARY[6,10]

- The infraclavicular block is carried out below the clavicle at the midpoint of the cord level of the brachial plexus.
- The improved safety is accorded by ultrasound guidance and less association with pneumothorax.
- Infraclavicular block can be a good substitute for supraclavicular and axillary blocks below the shoulder, and with advances, new techniques and approaches are being discovered with enhanced benefit of infraclavicular blocks.

REFERENCES

1. Hsu AC, Tai YT, Lin KH. Yao HY, Chiang HL, Ho BY, et al. Infraclavicular brachial plexus block in adults: a comprehensive review based on a unified nomenclature system. J Anesth. 2019;33: 463-77.
2. Klaastad Ø, Smith HJ, Smedby Ö, Winther-Larssen EH, Brodal P, Breivik H, et al. A novel infraclavicular brachial plexus block: the lateral and sagittal technique, developed by magnetic resonance imaging studies. Anesth Analg. 2004;98(1):252-6.
3. Raj PP, Montgomery SJ, Nettles D, Jenkins MT. Infraclavicular brachial plexus block—a new approach. Anesth Analg. 1973;52(6):897-904.
4. Scanaill PO, Valchev G. Ultrasound-Guided Infraclavicular Brachial Plexus Block.
5. Sims JK. A modification of landmarks for infraclavicular approach to brachial plexus block. Anesth Analg. 1977;56(4):554-5.
6. Williams LM, Singh K, Dua A, Singh A, Cummings A. Infraclavicular Nerve Block. In: StatPearls. StatPearls Publishing, Treasure Island (FL); 2025.
7. Chin KJ, Alakkad H, Adhikary SD, Singh M. Infraclavicular brachial plexus block for regional anaesthesia of the lower arm. Cochrane Database Syst Rev. 2013; 2013(8):CD005487.
8. Neuburger M, Kaiser H, Ass B, Franke C, Maurer H. Vertikale infraklavikuläre Plexus-brachialis-Blockade (VIP). Eine modifizierte Methode zur Optimierung der Punktionsortbestimmung unter Berücksichtigung des Pneumothoraxrisikos [Vertical infraclavicular blockade of the brachial plexus (VIP). A modified method to verify the puncture point under consideration of the risk of pneumothorax]. Anaesthesist. 2003;52(7):619-24.
9. Beh ZY, Hasan MS. Ultrasound-guided costoclavicular approach infraclavicular brachial plexus block for vascular access surgery. J Vasc Access. 2017;18(5):e57-61.
10. Stav A, Reytman L, Stav MY, Portnoy I, Kantarovsky A, Galili O, et al. Comparison of the Supraclavicular, Infraclavicular and Axillary Approaches for Ultrasound-Guided Brachial Plexus Block for Surgical Anesthesia. Rambam Maimonides Med J. 2016;7(2)e0013.
11. Sandhu NS, Capan LM. Ultrasound-guided infraclavicular brachial plexus block. Br J Anaesth. 2002;89(2):254-9.
12. Tran DQ, Boezaart AP, Neal JM. Beyond Ultrasound Guidance for Regional Anesthesiology. Reg Anesth Pain Med. 2017;42(5):556-63.
13. Sala-Blanch X, Reina MA, Pangthipampai P, Karmakar MK. Anatomic Basis for Brachial Plexus Block at the Costoclavicular Space: A Cadaver Anatomic Study. Reg Anesth Pain Med. 2016;41(3): 387-91.
14. Sharma D, Srivastava N, Pawar S, Garg R, Nagpal VK. Infraclavicular brachial plexus block: comparison of posterior cord stimulation with lateral or medial cord stimulation, a prospective double blinded study. Saudi J Anaesth. 2013;7(2):134-7.
15. Songthamwat B, Karmakar MK, Li JW, Samy W, Mok LYH. Ultrasound-Guided Infraclavicular Brachial Plexus Block: Prospective Randomized Comparison of the Lateral Sagittal and Costoclavicular Approach. Reg Anesth Pain Med. 2018;43(8):825-31.
16. Kavrut Ozturk N, Kavakli AS. Comparison of the coracoid and retroclavicular approaches for ultrasound-guided infraclavicular brachial plexus block. J Anesth. 2017;31(4):572-8.
17. Greher M, Retzl G, Niel P, Kamolz L, Marhofer P, Kapral S. Ultrasonographic assessment of topographic anatomy in volunteers suggests a modification of the infraclavicular vertical brachial plexus block. Br J Anaesth. 2002;88(5):632-6.
18. Leurcharusmee P, Elgueta MF, Tiyaprasertkul W, Sotthisopha T, Samerchua A, Gordon A, et al. A randomized comparison between costoclavicular and paracoracoid ultrasound-guided infraclavicular block for upper limb surgery. Can J Anaesth. 2017;64(6):617-25.

CHAPTER 5

Axillary Block

INTRODUCTION

An axillary approach to the brachial plexus nerve block was first introduced by Dr Halsted et al. in 1984, as even before introduction of ultrasound guidance this approach was useful in upper extremity surgeries.[1-4] This regional anesthesia technique blocks the brachial plexus terminal branches, i.e., radial, axillary, musculocutaneous, median, and ulnar at the axillary level. Unlike the inter scalene and infraclavicular and infraclavicular blocks, the risk of injury to stellate ganglion, pneumothorax, and diaphragmatic palsy are practically nonexistent with this block.[4,5]

IMPORTANT ANATOMICAL CONSIDERATIONS

The brachial plexus arises from the ventral rami of C5–C8, and at the level of the scalene muscles form the three trunks (superior, middle, and inferior) after leaving the inter scalene space they form two divisions (anterior and posterior) at the supraclavicular level. At the infraclavicular level division regroup into three cords (lateral, posterior, and medial) and finally at the axillary level five terminal branches (radial, axillary, musculocutaneous, median, and ulnar) at the lateral border of the pectoralis minor muscle.[4-7]

The median nerve is formed from lateral and medial cords, the musculocutaneous nerve is formed from lateral cord, the ulnar from medial cord, and the axillary and radial nerves from the posterior cord.

INDICATIONS[4,8]

- Surgery of elbow, forearm, wrist, and hand
- Postoperative pain control for upper extremity surgeries
- Complex regional pain syndrome of upper extremity

CONTRAINDICATIONS[4,5]

- *Absolute:*
    - Local anesthetic allergy
    - Patient refusal
    - Infection at the local site
    - Lack of skilled assistance
    - Lack of resuscitation equipment
- *Relative:*
    - Deranged coagulation
    - Systemic infection

EQUIPMENT[4,5]

Healthcare professionals performing infraclavicular block should be equipped with the following items:

- Standard physiological monitors [electrocardiogram (ECG), BP apparatus, and pulse oximeter]
- Resuscitation equipment
- Ultrasound machine with a high frequency linear transducer (8–15 MHz)
- Sterile gloves, drapes, and ultrasonography (USG) probe covers
- Skin antiseptics, e.g., betadine, alcohol, and chlorhexidine

- Local anesthetic, i.e., 2% lidociane
- Mild sedative agents, i.e., 1–2 mg of midazolam
- Regional block local anesthesia (0.5% bupivacaine/ropivacaine for postoperative analgesia and 2% lidocaine for short onset time requirement)
- Short bevel insulated, stimulating block needle 50 mm (22-gauge for single injection and 18 gauge for continuous catheter), insulated, stimulating needle
- A 3-mL syringe with a 25-gauge needle with local anesthetic agent for skin infiltration
- One 10–20 mL syringe with local anesthetic
- Marking pen

PERSONNEL

The infraclavicular block requires two persons, one to control the ultrasound probe and needle, other to manage the syringe and inject local anesthetic. Additional person will monitor the vitals of the patient and will administer the emergency drugs if needed.[4,5]

ULTRASOUND-GUIDED AXILLARY BLOCK TECHNIQUE

- The provider must perform the process of informed consent.
- Gain intravenous access, apply standard monitors, and perform standard safety checklist.
- *Patient positioning*: The patient can be positioned in supine position with arms 90° of abduction and flexed at the elbow to have optimal relationship of landmarks to the brachial plexus.[4,8]
- Mild sedation with 1–2 mg of midazolam may be provided though many patients do not need it.[1]
- Skin antiseptic is applied to the skin, then sterile conduction gel is applied to the ultrasound transducer and use of sterile probe cover is recommended.[1,2] The block can be performed awake or under sedation.[9]
- *Transducer positioning and technique:*[4,7,8-15] The high frequency linear transducer is placed over the axillary fold in the transverse axis. The important structure to visualize while performing the USG-guided infraclavicular block of brachial plexus is axillary artery seen lying over the conjoined tendon of latissimus dorsi and teres major muscle tendons. It is seen as dark, round, pulsating structure with hyperechoic walls, axillary vein lying beside the artery, which is compressible and collapsible, the confirmation can be made on color Doppler. The median, ulnar, and radial nerves are seen around the artery seen as honeycomb structure of variable echogenicity. The median nerve lies at 11 o'clock, ulnar nerve at 2 o'clock, and radial nerve at 5–6 o'clock position. The musculocutaneous nerve is seen more distally in the upper arm a few centimeters away from the axilla lying between coracobrachialis and biceps brachii, seen classically as triangular shaped **(Figs. 1A and B)**. Once the structure is identified, then 50 mm 22G short bevel needle is advanced in plane under ultrasound guidance through locally anesthetized skin. The syringe aspiration is done to rule out intravascular location and the local anesthetic is injected the deposition of anesthetic is obtained around the nerve by hydrodissection method. The hydrodissection technique help in nerve identification, and it also moves the nerve away from the vessels. Three types of injecting techniques are employed:
    1. Single injection
    2. Dual injection
    3. Multiple injections

The time of onset of axillary block varies according to these techniques and on an average, it is 10.2 minutes.

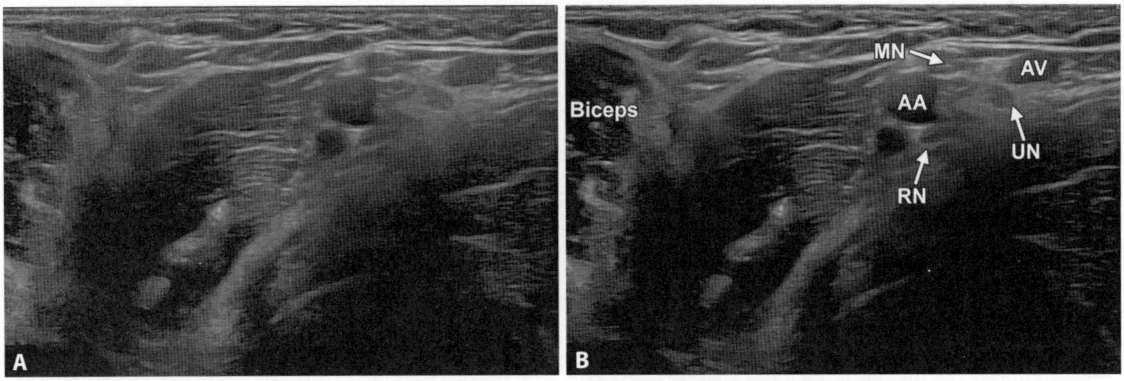

Figs. 1A and B: Sonographic anatomy of axillary fossa from superficial to deep with terminal nerves of brachial plexus, i.e., median nerve (MN), ulnar nerve (UN) and radial nerve (RN) seen around the axillar artery (AA) and axillary vein (AV).

SIDE EFFECTS[14]

- Temporary numbness and weakness
- Discomfort at injection site

COMPLICATIONS[14-16]

- Infection
- Bleeding/hematoma
- Local anesthetic toxicity
- Vascular puncture
- Intravascular toxicity
- Needle-induced paresthesia
- Permanent nerve injury

SUMMARY[17-19]

- The axillary nerve block is technically easy and used in high degree of success in upper limb surgeries and procedures.
- The improved safety as there is less association with pneumothorax and phrenic nerve injury.

REFERENCES

1. de Jong RH. Axillary block of the brachial plexus. Anesthesiology. 1961;22:215-25.
2. Bosomworth PP, Egbert LD, Hamelberg W. Block of the brachial plexus in the axilla: its value and complications. Ann Surg. 1961;154(6):911-4.
3. Orebaugh SL, Williams BA. Brachial plexus anatomy: normal and variant. Sci World J. 2009;9:300-12.
4. Janjua MS, Pak A. Axillary Block. [Updated 2023 Jun 20]. In: StatPearls [Internet]. Treasure Island (FL): StatPearls Publishing; 2025 Jan. Available from: https://www.ncbi.nlm.nih.gov/books/NBK537201/
5. Wingate R, Foxall G, Russon K. Ultrasound Guided Axillary Brachial Plexus Block. Anaesth Tutor Week. 2016;4(2).
6. Strub B, Sonderegger J, Campe AV, Grünert J, Osterwalder JJ. What benefits does ultrasound-guided axillary block for brachial plexus anaesthesia offer over the conventional blind approach in hand surgery? J Hand Surg (European Volume). 2011;36(9):778-86.
7. Lopera-Velásquez LM, Restrepo-Garcés C. Ultrasound and nerve stimulation-guided axillary block. Colomb J Anesth. 2016;44(1):30-5.
8. Gili S, Abreo A, GóMez-Fernández M, Solà R, Morros C, Sala-Blanch X. Patterns of Distribution of the Nerves Around the Axillary Artery Evaluated by Ultrasound and Assessed by Nerve Stimulation During Axillary Block. Clin Anat. 2019;32(1):2-8.
9. Silva MG, Sala-Blanch X, Marin R, Espinoza X, Arauz A, Morros C. Bloqueo axilar ecoguiado: variaciones anatómicas de la disposición de los 4 nervios terminales del plexo braquial en relación con la arteria humeral. Revista Española de Anestesiología y Reanimación. 2014;61(1):15-20.

10. Wada T, Yamauchi M, Oki G, Sonoda T, Yamakage M, Yamashita T. Efficacy of axillary nerve block in elbow arthroscopic surgery: a randomized trial. Journal of shoulder and elbow surgery. 2014;23(3):291-6.
11. Ustuner E, Yılmaz A, Özgencil E, Okten F, Turhan SC. Ultrasound anatomy of the brachial plexus nerves in the neurovascular bundle at the axilla in patients undergoing upper-extremity block anesthesia. Skeletal Radiol. 2013;42:707-13.
12. Duger C, Isbir AC, Kaygusuz K, Kol IO, Gursoy S, Ozturk H, et al. The importance of needle echogenity in ultrasound guided axillary brachial plexus block: a randomized controlled clinical study. Int J Med Sci. 2013;10(9):1108.
13. Vassiliou T, Müller HH, Ellert A, Wallot P, Kwee KM, Beyerle M, et al. High-versus low-stimulation current threshold for axillary plexus blocks: a prospective randomized triple-blinded noninferiority trial in 205 patients. Anesth Analg. 2013;116(1):247-54.
14. Nadeau MJ, Lévesque S, Dion N. Ultrasound-guided regional anesthesia for upper limb surgery. Can J Anesth. 2013;60(3):304.
15. Cho S, Kim YJ, Kim JH, Baik HJ. Double-injection perivascular ultrasound-guided axillary brachial plexus block according to needle positioning: 12 versus 6 o'clock position of the axillary artery. Korean J Anesth. 2014;66(2):112-9.
16. López-Morales S, Moreno-Martín A, del Ojo JL, Rodriguez-Huertas F. Bloqueo axilar ecoguiado frente a bloqueo infraclavicular ecoguiado para la cirugía de miembro superior. Revista Española de Anestesiología y Reanimación. 2013;60(6): 313-9.
17. Sariguney D, Mahli A, Coskun D. The extent of blockade following axillary and infraclavicular approaches of brachial plexus block in uremic patients. J Clin Med Res. 2012;4(1):26.
18. Satapathy AR, Coventry DM. Axillary brachial plexus block. Anesthesiol Res Pract. 2011;2011: 173796.
19. Zhu W, Zhou R, Chen L, Chen Y, Huang L, Xia Y, et al. The ultrasound-guided selective nerve block in the upper arm: an approach of retaining the motor function in elbow. BMC Anesthesiol. 2018;18(1):143.

SECTION 3

Truncal and Neural Axial Blocks

CHAPTER 6

Thoracic Paravertebral Block

INTRODUCTION

Thoracic paravertebral block (TPVB) is a technique to inject local anesthetic in the paravertebral location from where the spinal nerves exit the intervertebral foramen. Hugo sellheim first pioneered this block in 1905, which is widely used in clinical practice nowadays to provide unilateral, segmental, somatic, and sympathetic nerve block at multiple vertebral levels.[1,2] It has implication in management of pain of unilateral origin from chest or abdomen as well as surgical anesthesia of thorax.[3,4]

IMPORTANT ANATOMICAL CONSIDERATIONS[5-7]

The paravertebral space is a wedge-shaped potential compartment seen bilaterally on the side of vertebral bodies having structures at the boundaries as:

- Anterolateral-partial pleura
- Posterior-superior costotransverse ligament
- Medial-vertebrae and intervertebral foramina
- Superior-inferior aspect of rib head
- Inferior- superior aspect of rib head
- As the paravertebral space has endothoracic fascia, it devised further into anterior and posterior compartments.

INDICATIONS[5,6]

- Analgesia (rib fractures, refractory angina, cancer pain, and complex regional pain syndrome)
- Anesthesia and analgesia in hemithorax surgical procedure
- Perioperative bilateral TPBV thoracic phase of major abdominal surgeries.

CONTRAINDICATIONS[7,8]

- *Absolute:*
  - Local anesthetic allergy
  - Patient refusal
  - Infection at the local paraspinal site
  - Lack of skilled assistance
  - Lack of resuscitation equipment
- *Relative:*
  - Deranged coagulation
  - Systemic infection
  - Diaphragmatic palsy
  - Severe respiratory disease

EQUIPMENT[9,10]

Healthcare professionals performing infraclavicular block should be equipped with the following items:

- Standard physiological monitors [electrocardiogram (ECG), BP apparatus, and pulse oximeter]
- Resuscitation equipment
- Ultrasound machine with a curvilinear or linear transducer
- Sterile gloves, drapes, and ultrasonography (USG) probe covers
- Skin antiseptics, e.g., betadine, alcohol, and chlorhexidine
- Local anesthetic, i.e., 2% lidociane
- Mild sedative agents, i.e., 1–2 mg of midazolam
- Regional block local anesthesia 20–30 mL (0.25% bupivacaine/0.2 ropivacaine for postoperative analgesia)

- Short bevel insulated, stimulating block needle 80 mm B-level nerve block needle
- A 3-mL syringe with a 25-gauge needle with local anesthetic agent for skin infiltration
- One 20 mL syringe with local anesthetic
- Marking pen

PERSONNEL

The thoracic paravertebral block requires two persons, one to control the ultrasound probe and needle, other to manage the syringe and inject local anesthetic. Additional person will monitor the vitals of the patient and will administer the emergency drugs if needed[1,10]

ULTRASONOGRAPHY-GUIDED THORACIC PARAVERTEBRAL BLOCK TECHNIQUE[4,10,11]

- The provider must perform the process of informed consent.
- Gain intravenous access, apply standard monitors, and perform standard safety check list.
- *Patient positioning:* The patient can be positioned in seated, lateral, or prone; however, the seated position is more comfortable, especially in awake patient. The clinician performing the block and ultrasound machine should be placed ergonomically.

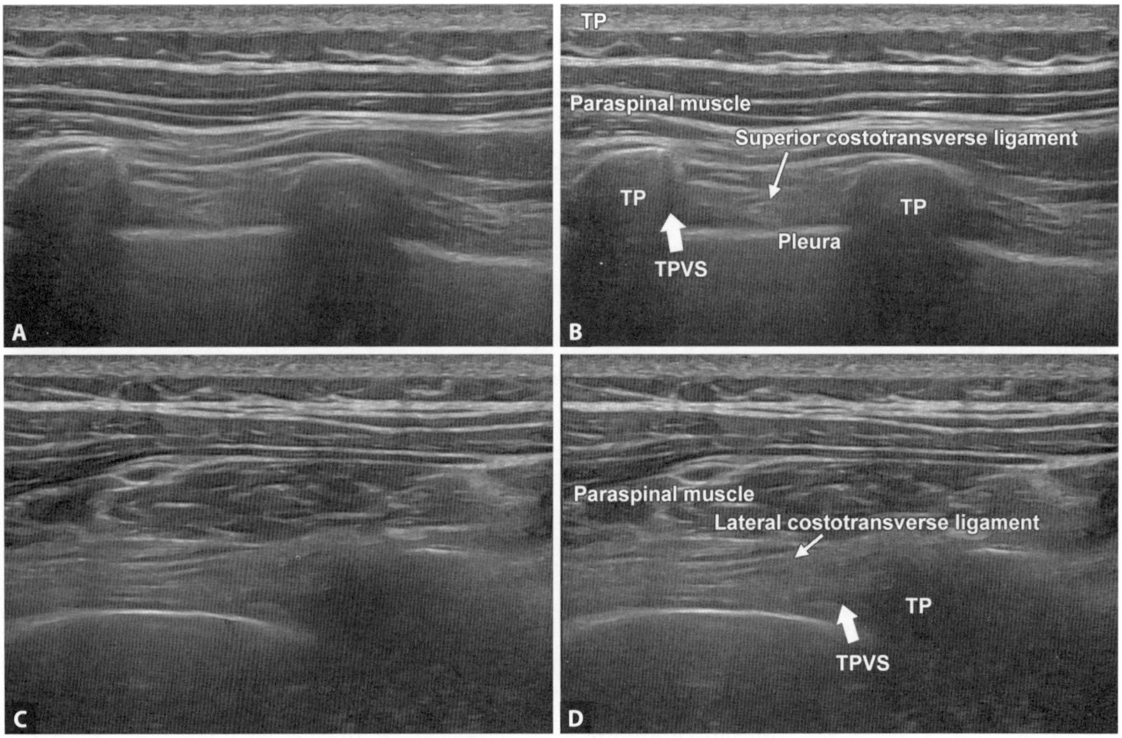

Figs. 1A to D: A and B (*parasagittal*) show the thoracic paravertebral space (TPVS) seen (white thick arrow) between the superior costotransverse ligament (white thin arrow) and parietal pleura. C and D (*transverse*) show sonographic anatomy when the beam is insinuated between two transverse processes and superficial to deep plane is seen which is showing thoracic paravertebral space, which is seen by hypoechoic area (white thick arrow) between the lateral costotransverse ligament and pleura (white thin arrow).

- Mild sedation with 1–2 mg of midazolam may be provided though many patients do not need it.
- Skin antiseptic is applied to the skin, then sterile conduction gel is applied to the ultrasound transducer and use of sterile probe cover is recommended. The block can be performed awake or under sedation.
- *Transducer positioning and technique:*[12-14] After identifying the spinous processes by landmark based on C1 vertebra and lower edge of scapula identification (which corresponds to T7). The ultrasound transducer is placed on the spinous processes as per desires surgical plane, then on lateral moving the probe the transverse process is identified and moving the probe oblique three anatomical structures are visualized (**Figs. 1A to D**):
  1. Internal intercostal membrane
  2. Transverse process
  3. Parietal pleura

In the locally anesthetized skin, the needle tip is traversed by in plane technique with intermittent aspiration to avoid vascular access and when the tip reaches in the space between intercostal membrane and the pleura local anesthetic is administered slowly over 30 seconds.

SIDE EFFECTS[1,10]

- Infection
- Nerve injury
- Allergic reaction
- Local anesthetic toxicity

COMPLICATIONS[15]

- Epidural/intrathecal spread
- Epidural placement
- Paravertebral muscle pain
- Pleural puncture
- Pneumothorax
- Vessel puncture
- Bleeding/hematoma
- Failed block

SUMMARY

- The TPVB is done for somatosensory and sympathetic nerve block at multiple vertebral levels.
- As pneumothorax is a serious complication of the block real time depression of pleura during local anesthetic under ultrasound guidance is an indication of correct placement of needle tip in the paravertebral space.

REFERENCES

1. Karmakar MK. Thoracic paravertebral block. Anesthesiology. 2001;95(3):771-80.
2. Richardson J, Lönnqvist PA. Thoracic paravertebral block. Br J Anaesth. 1998;81(2):230-8.
3. Cheema SP, Ilsley D, Richardson J, Sabanathan S. A thermographic study of paravertebral analgesia. Anaesthesia. 1995;50(2):118-21.
4. Saito T, Den S, Cheema SP, Tanuma K, Carney E, Carlsson C, et al. A single-injection, multisegmental paravertebral block-extension of somatosensory and sympathetic block in volunteers. Acta Anaesthesiol Scand. 2001;45(1): 30-3.
5. Kurian J. Single injection paravertebral block. Acta Anaesthesiol Scand. 2001;45(8):1055.
6. Conacher ID. Resin injection of thoracic paravertebral spaces. Br J Anaesth. 1988;61(6): 657-61.
7. Cowie B, McGlade D, Ivanusic J, Barrington MJ. Ultrasound-guided thoracic paravertebral blockade: a cadaveric study. Anesth Analg. 2010; 110(6):1735-9.
8. Richardson J, Vowden P, Sabanathan S. Bilateral paravertebral analgesia for major abdominal vascular surgery: a preliminary report. Anaesthesia. 1995;50(11):995-8.
9. Zheng C, Wang J, Xie S. Ultrasound-Guided Thoracic Paravertebral Nerve Block on Postoperative Pain, Quality of Life, and Recovery in Patients with Non-Small-Cell Lung Cancer. Biomed Res Int. 2021;2021:6692815.
10. Ben Aziz M, Mukhdomi J. Thoracic Paravertebral Block. In: StatPearls. Treasure Island (FL): StatPearls Publishing; 2025.

11. Hu L, Xu X, Tian H, He J. Effect of Single-Injection Thoracic Paravertebral Block via the Intrathoracic Approach for Analgesia After Single-Port Video-Assisted Thoracoscopic Lung Wedge Resection: A Randomized Controlled Trial. Pain Ther. 2021;10(1):433-42.
12. Luyet C, Eichenberger U, Greif R, Vogt A, Szücs Farkas Z, Moriggl B. Ultrasound-guided paravertebral puncture and placement of catheters in human cadavers: an imaging study. Br J Anaesth. 2009;102(4):534-9.
13. Jones A, Le-Wendling L, Ihnatsenka B, Smith C, Baker E, Boezaart A. Empirical guide to a safe thoracic paravertebral block based on dimensions of paravertebral space when ultrasound visualization is challenging. Reg Anesth Pain Med. 2024;49(2):133-8.
14. Krediet AC, Moayeri N, van Geffen GJ, Bruhn J, Renes S, Bigeleisen PE, et al. Different Approaches to Ultrasound-guided Thoracic Paravertebral Block: An Illustrated Review. Anesthesiology. 2015;123(2):459-74.
15. Riain SC, Donnell BO, Cuffe T, Harmon DC, Fraher JP, Shorten G. Thoracic paravertebral block using real-time ultrasound guidance. Anesth Analg. 2010;110(1):248-51.

CHAPTER 7

Erector Spinae Plane Block

INTRODUCTION

The erector spinae plane block is an interfacial paraspinal plane block regional anesthesia technique used to provide analgesia for variety of surgeries and pain alleviation procedures. This technique was first used by Forero et al. in patients with severe chronic thoracis neuropathic pain and is now commonly used in a variety of thoracic and trunk surgeries.[1,2]

IMPORTANT ANATOMICAL CONSIDERATIONS

With the aim of spread of local anesthetic as compartmental spread and blocking the dorsal as well as ventral rami of the spinal nerves which gives a multi-dermatomal sensory block to thoracic and abdominal walls.[3,4] The erector spinae block is most often performed in the T5-T7 paraspinal levels but can be performed at caudal levels too.

INDICATIONS[5,6]

- Spine surgery
- Rib fractures
- Thoracic surgery—postlateral thoracotomy analgesia
- Breast surgery
- Cardiac surgery
- Lower limb surgery
- Anorectal surgery

CONTRAINDICATIONS[7,8]

- *Absolute:*
    - Local anesthetic allergy
    - Patient refusal
    - Infection at the local paraspinal site
    - Lack of skilled assistance
    - Lack of resuscitation equipment
- *Relative:*
    - Deranged coagulation
    - Systemic infection

EQUIPMENT[3,4,8]

Healthcare professionals performing infraclavicular block should be equipped with the following items:

- Standard physiological monitors [electrocardiogram (ECG), BP apparatus, and pulse oximeter]
- Resuscitation equipment
- Ultrasound machine with a linear transducer (6–12 MHz)
- Sterile gloves, drapes, and ultrasonography (USG) probe covers
- Skin antiseptics, e.g., betadine, alcohol, and chlorhexidine
- Local anesthetic, i.e., 2% lidociane
- Mild sedative agents, i.e., 1–2 mg of midazolam
- Regional block local anesthesia 20–30 mL (0.25% bupivacaine/0.2 ropivacaine for postoperative analgesia)
- Short bevel insulated, stimulating block needle 50–100 mm (22-gauge for single injection and 18-gauge Tuohy needle for continuous infusion) and an epidural catheter (in case of continuous infusion)
- A 3-mL syringe with a 25-gauge needle with local anesthetic agent for skin infiltration
- One 20-mL syringe with local anesthetic
- Marking pen

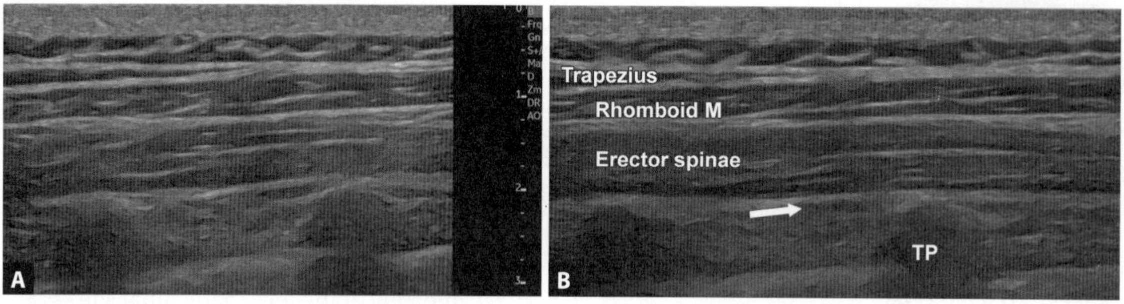

Figs. 1A and B: Sonographic anatomy of erector spinae plane from superficial to deep and arrow indicating the target site for local anesthetic spread deep into erector spinae muscle.

PERSONNEL

The Erector spinae plane block requires two persons, one to control the ultrasound probe and needle, other to manage the syringe and inject local anesthetic. Additional person will monitor the vitals of the patient and will administer the emergency drugs if needed.

ULTRASONOGRAPHY-GUIDED ERECTOR SPINAE PLANE BLOCK TECHNIQUE[4,9-11]

- The provider must perform the process of informed consent.
- Gain intravenous access, apply standard monitors, and perform standard safety check list.
- *Patient positioning*: The patient can be positioned in prone and the clinician performing the block and ultrasound machine should be placed ergonomically.
- Mild sedation with 1–2 mg of midazolam may be provided though many patients do not need it.
- Skin antiseptic is applied to the skin, then sterile conduction gel is applied to the ultrasound transducer, and use of sterile probe cover is recommended. The block can be performed awake or under sedation.
- *Transducer positioning and technique:*[4,6,12] The linear transducer should be placed in a cephalocaudal direction in the midline at desired level, then moved laterally and transverse processes are identified. superficial to the transverse process at the higher thoracic levels, i.e., above T5, the trapezius, rhomboid major, and erector spinae are identified in layers whereas in lower and mid-thorax level, only trapezius and erector spinae are visualized **(Figs. 1A and B)**. The Tuohy needle tip after anesthetizing the skin should be inserted by in-plane technique from cephalad to caudal direction till it reaches the transverse process first 1–2 mL of local anesthetic is injected under ultrasound guidance and its spread superficial to transverse process and deep to erector spinae is seen. On confirmation under frequent aspiration nerve block is completed by injecting 20–30 mL of local anesthetic.

SIDE EFFECTS[6,13]

- Discomfort at injection site
- Infection at needle insertion site

COMPLICATIONS[4]

- Local anesthetic toxicity
- Pleural puncture
- Pneumothorax
- Vessel puncture
- Bleeding/hematoma
- Failed block

SUMMARY

- Erector spinae plane block is multimodal analgesia is an effective and safely performable plane block having distinctive advantage in large number of indications.
- It is relatively a simple and effective technique for the management of perioperative pain.

REFERENCES

1. Forero M, Adhikary SD, Lopez H, Tsui C, Chin KJ. The erector spinae plane block: a novel analgesic technique in thoracic neuropathic pain. Reg Anesth Pain Med. 2016;41(5):621-7.
2. Krishnan S, Cascella M. Erector Spinae Plane Block. In: StatPearls. StatPearls Publishing, Treasure Island (FL); 2023.
3. Yoshizaki M, Murata H, Ogami-Takamura K, Hara T. Bilateral erector spinae plane block using a programmed intermittent bolus technique for pain management after Nuss procedure. J Clin Anesth. 2019;57:51-52.
4. Raft J, Chin KJ, Belanger ME, Clairoux A, Richebé P, Brulotte V. Continuous erector spinae plane block for thoracotomy analgesia after epidural failure. J Clin Anesth. 2019;54:132-3.
5. Chin KJ, Adhikary S, Sarwani N, Forero M. The analgesic efficacy of pre-operative bilateral erector spinae plane (ESP) blocks in patients having ventral hernia repair. Anaesthesia. 2017;72(4):452-60.
6. Pawa A, King C, Thang C, White L. Erector spinae plane block: the ultimate 'plan A'block? Br J Anaesth. 2023;130(5):497-502.
7. Chin KJ, Lewis S. Opioid-free Analgesia for Posterior Spinal Fusion Surgery Using Erector Spinae Plane (ESP) Blocks in a Multimodal Anesthetic Regimen. Spine (Phila Pa 1976). 2019; 44(6):E379-83.
8. Oostvogels L, Weibel S, Meißner M, Kranke P, Meyer-Frießem CH, Pogatzki-Zahn E, et al. Erector spinae plane block for postoperative pain. Cochrane Database Syst Rev. 2024;2: CD013763.
9. Pourkashanian A, Narayanan M, Venkataraju A. The erector spinae plane block: a review of current evidence. Update Anaesth. 2020;35: 27-33.
10. Zhang J, He Y, Wang S, Chen Z, Zhang Y, Gao Y, et al. The erector spinae plane block causes only cutaneous sensory loss on ipsilateral posterior thorax: a prospective observational volunteer study. BMC Anesthesiol. 2020;20(1):88.
11. Forero M, Rajarathinam M, Adhikary S, Chin KJ. Erector spinae plane (ESP) block in the management of post thoracotomy pain syndrome: a case series. Scand J Pain. 2017;17: 325-9.
12. Zengin, SU, Ergun, MO & Gunal, O. Effect of Ultrasound-Guided Erector Spinae Plane Block on Postoperative Pain and Intraoperative Opioid Consumption in Bariatric Surgery. OBES SURG 31, 5176–5182 (2021). https://doi.org/10.1007/s11695-021-05681-7
13. Bugada D, Zarcone AG, Manini M, Lorini LF. Continuous Erector Spinae Block at lumbar level (L4) for prolonged postoperative analgesia after hip surgery. J Clin Anesth. 2019;52:24-25. doi: 10.1016/j.jclinane.2018.08.023. Epub 2018 Aug 25. PMID: 30153539

CHAPTER 8

Rectus Sheath Block

INTRODUCTION

The rectus sheath block which is used to facilitate surgery involving anterior abdominal wall was first described by Schleich in 1989.[1] The rectus sheath block done unilaterally and bilaterally is given to provide pain relief after surgeries in midline abdominal surgeries. Under the guidance of ultrasound, the risk of vascular injury is very less making the technique safe and popular.[2,3]

IMPORTANT ANATOMICAL CONSIDERATIONS

The ventral rami of the thoracolumbar spinal segmental nerve (T7-L1) innervate the anterior abdominal wall; these branches reach the rectus muscle near the midline after coursing between the rectus abdominis muscle and the rectus sheath. Even single injection of local anesthetic injection is spread craniocaudally within this compartment because the tendinous insertions of the rectus muscle are not fused to the posterior rectus sheath.[2,4,5]

INDICATIONS[6]

- Hernia repair (umbilical, paraumbilical, and epigastric)
- Pyloromyotomy
- Laparoscopic surgery
- Abdominoplasty

CONTRAINDICATIONS[3]

- *Absolute:*
  - Local anesthetic allergy
  - Patient refusal
  - Infection at the local site
  - Lack of skilled assistance
  - Lack of resuscitation equipment
- *Relative:*
  - Deranged coagulation
  - Systemic infection

EQUIPMENT[3,4,7]

Healthcare professionals performing infraclavicular block should be equipped with the following items:

- Standard physiological monitors [electrocardiogram (ECG), BP apparatus, and pulse oximeter)
- Resuscitation equipment
- Ultrasound machine with a linear transducer (2–5 MHz)
- Sterile gloves, drapes, and ultrasonography (USG) probe covers
- Skin antiseptics, e.g., betadine, alcohol, and chlorhexidine
- Local anesthetic, i.e., 2% lidociane
- Mild sedative agents, i.e., 1–2 mg of midazolam
- Regional block local anesthesia (0.25% bupivacaine, 0.2% ropivacaine 2% lidociane for postoperative analgesia)
- Short bevel insulated, stimulating block needle 50–100 mm (22-gauge for single injection and 18 gauge for continuous catheter), insulated, stimulating needle
- A 3-mL syringe with a 25-gauge needle with local anesthetic agent for skin infiltration
- One 20-mL syringe with local anesthetic
- Marking pen

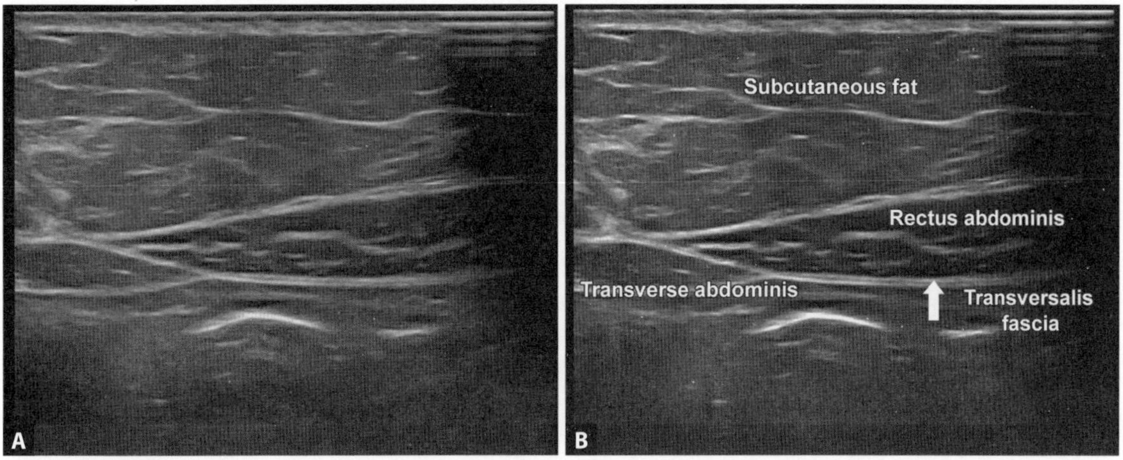

Figs. 1A and B: Sonographic anatomy of transverse plane from superficial to deep and labeled anatomical structures. The arrow indicating the injectate local anesthetic spread should be between the posterior rectus sheath and transversalis fascia.

PERSONNEL

The rectus sheath block requires two persons, one to control the ultrasound probe and needle, other to manage the syringe and inject local anesthetic. Additional person will monitor the vitals of the patient and will administer the emergency drugs if needed.[4,8]

ULTRASONOGRAPHY-GUIDED SUPRAUMBILICAL TECHNIQUE[4,9]

- The provider must perform the process of informed consent.
- Gain intravenous access, apply standard monitors, and perform standard safety check list.
- *Patient positioning:* The patient can be positioned in supine and the clinician performing the block and ultrasound machine should be placed ergonomically.
- Mild sedation with 1–2 mg of midazolam may be provided though many patients do not need it.
- Skin antiseptic is applied to the skin, then sterile conduction gel is applied to the ultrasound transducer and use of sterile probe cover is recommended. The block can be performed awake or under sedation.
- *Transducer positioning and technique (**Figs. 1A and B**):* The linear ultrasound transducer should be placed just above the umbilicus in transverse direction at the midline with depth selection made as per the abdominal wall thickness. Now move the plane laterally rectus muscle is visualized and if moved more laterally lateral border of semilunaris muscle is visualized. The tip insertion is seen in plane of the ultrasound beam and as the intercostal nerve traverse the abdominal wall in between the internal oblique and transverse abdominis, they enter the posterior rectus sheath. These nerves traverse through the belly and posterior rectus sheath to the midline.[10,11] The needle is routed between rectus sheath and posterior rectus sheath in the lateral aspect of rectus sheath. Thus, local anesthetic is injected with regular aspirations to avoid intravascular injection here, with advantage of nonfusion of tendinous intersections of posterior rectus sheath which allows local spread beyond compartments. Commonly 0.2% ropivacaine

in dose of 3 mg/kg is limited in children and in adults 10–15 mL of volume is given.[4,12]

SIDE EFFECT[2]

Discomfort at injection site.

COMPLICATIONS[4]

- Peritoneal puncture
- Perforation of the bowel
- Visceral puncture
- Vessel puncture
- Retroperitoneal bleeding/hematoma

SUMMARY

- A rectus sheath block enables intraoperative and postoperative analgesia for mid-line abdominal surgeries.
- A shallow trajectory should be ensured.

REFERENCES

1. Schleich DL. Schmerzlose Operationen, 4th edition. Berlin: Springer Verlag; 1899; pp. 240-58.
2. Snell R. Clinical Anatomy, 8th edition. Baltimore: Lippincott Williams & Wilkins; 2008.
3. Abrahams MS, Horn JL, Noles LM, Aziz MF. Evidence-based medicine: ultrasound guidance for truncal blocks. Reg Anesth Pain Med. 2010;35(Suppl 2):S36-42.
4. Kwon HJ, Kim YJ, Kim Y, Kim S, Cho H, Lee JH, et al. Complications and technical consideration of ultrasound-guided rectus sheath blocks: a retrospective analysis of 4033 patients. Anesth Analg. 136(2):365-72.
5. Azemati S, Khosravi MB. An assessment of the value of rectus sheath block for postlaparoscopic pain in gynecologic surgery. J Minim Invasive Gynecol. 2005;12(1):12-5.
6. Cornish P, Deacon A. Rectus sheath catheters for continuous analgesia after upper abdominal surgery. ANZ J Surg. 2007;77(1-2):84.
7. Osaka Y, Kashiwagi M, Nagatsuka Y, Oosaku M, Hirose C. [Ultrasound-guided rectus sheath block for upper abdominal surgery]. Masui. 2010;59(8):1039-41.
8. Willschke H, Bösenberg A, Marhofer P, Johnston S, Kettner SC, Wanzel O, et al. Ultrasonography-guided rectus sheath block in paediatric anaesthesia—a new approach to an old technique. Br J Anaesth. 2006;97(2):244-9.
9. Sandeman DJ, Dilley AV. Ultrasound-guided rectus sheath block and catheter placement. ANZ J Surg. 2008;78(7):621-3.
10. Kartalov A, Jankulovski N, Kuzmanovska B, Zdravkovska M, Shosholcheva M, Tolevska M, et al. The effect of rectus sheath block as a supplement of general anesthesia on postoperative analgesia in adult patient undergoing umbilical hernia repair. Contributions, Sec Biol Med Sci 2018; 38(3):135-42.
11. Fuzier R. ALR échoguidée: les blocs de la paroi abdominale [Ultrasound-guided TAP, rectus sheath, ilioinguinal and ilio-hypogastric blocks]. Ann Fr Anesth Reanim. 2012;31(9):e207-9.
12. Husain NK, Ravalia A. Ultrasound-guided ilio-inguinal and rectus sheath nerve blocks. Anaesthesia. 2006;61(11):1126.

CHAPTER 9

Transverse Abdominis Plane Blocks

INTRODUCTION

The transverse abdominis plane (TAP) is a regional anesthetic block used for perioperative pain control of the anterior and lateral abdominal wall described first by Rafi et al. in 2001, and Hebbard et al. in 2007 described the technique ultrasound guidance.[1,2] The ultrasonography (USG)-guided techniques are considered the gold standard as it is easy to acquire images and is safe as performed under direct visualization.[3]

IMPORTANT ANATOMICAL CONSIDERATIONS

The transverse abdominis block is an effective regional anesthetic technique that blocks neural afferents of the T6-11 spinal nerves providing innervation to the anterior abdominal wall. It provides analgesia to the anterior and lateral abdominal wall by anesthetizing the intercostal, subcostal, iliohypogastric, and ilioinguinal nerves.[3,4]

INDICATIONS[3,5-8]

- *Unilateral:*
  - Appendicectomy
  - Cholecystectomy
  - Nephrectomy
  - Renal transplant
- *Bilateral block:*
  - Ventral hernia repair
  - Umbilical hernia repair
  - Cesarian delivery
  - Laparoscopic surgery

CONTRAINDICATIONS[3,8-10]

- *Absolute:*
  - Local anesthetic allergy
  - Patient refusal
  - Infection at the local site
  - Lack of skilled assistance
  - Lack of resuscitation equipment
- *Relative:*
  - Deranged coagulation
  - Systemic infection

EQUIPMENT[3,8,11]

Healthcare professionals performing infraclavicular block should be equipped with the following items:

- Standard physiological monitors [electrocardiogram (ECG), BP apparatus, and pulse oximeter)
- Resuscitation equipment
- Ultrasound machine with a high-frequency linear transducer (8–15 MHz)
- Sterile gloves, drapes, and USG probe covers
- Skin antiseptics, e.g., betadine, alcohol, and chlorhexidine
- Local anesthetic, i.e., 2% lidocaine
- Mild sedative agents, i.e., 1–2 mg of midazolam
- Regional block local anesthesia (0.25% bupivacaine, rest/0.2% ropivacaine/2% lidocaine for postoperative analgesia)
- Short bevel insulated, stimulating block needle 50–100 mm (20-22-gauge for single injection)

- A 5-mL syringe with a 25-gauge needle with local anesthetic agent for skin infiltration
- Two 20-mL syringes with local anesthetic
- Marking pen

PERSONNEL

The TAP block requires two persons, one to control the ultrasound probe and needle and other person will monitor the vitals of the patient and will administer the emergency drugs if needed.[3,12]

ULTRASONOGRAPHY GUIDED TRANSVERSE ABDOMINIS PLANE BLOCK TECHNIQUE[3,11]

- The provider must perform the process of informed consent.
- Gain intravenous access, apply standard monitors, and perform standard safety checklist.
- The preprocedural time out should occur before starting the procedure.

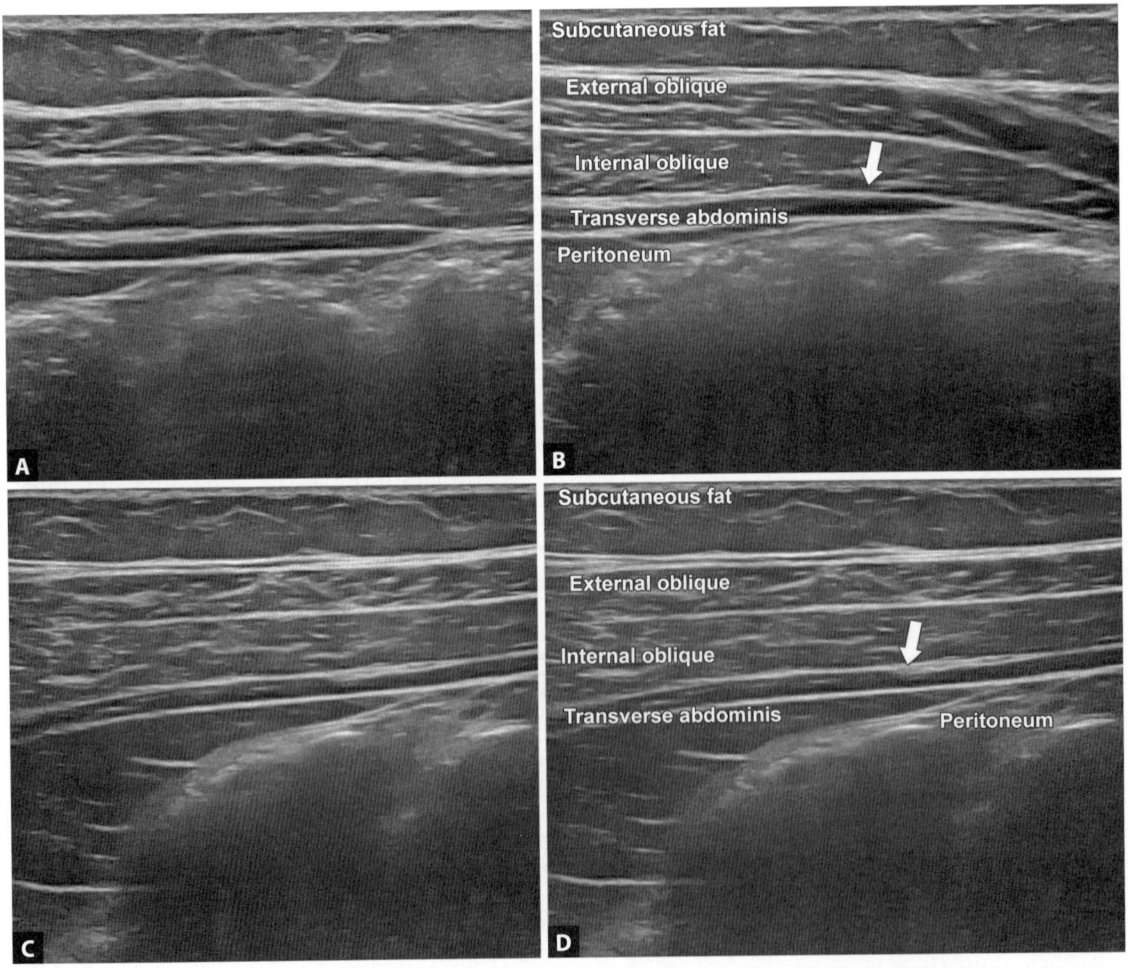

Figs. 1A to D: Sonographic anatomy of transverse plane from superficial to deep and labeled anatomical structures (B and D). The white arrow indicating the injectate local anesthetic spread should be between the internal oblique muscle and transverse abdominis muscle.

- *Patient positioning:* The patient can be positioned in supine position with uncovered abdomen.
- Mild sedation with 1–2 mg of midazolam may be provided though many patients do not need it.[3]
- Skin antiseptic is applied to the skin, then sterile conduction gel is applied to the ultrasound transducer and use of sterile probe cover is recommended. The block can be performed awake or under sedation.
- *Transducer positioning and technique:*[3, 4,11,13] The ultrasound-guided TAP block has three approaches as follows (**Figs. 1A to D**):
  1. *Subcostal approach* for anterior abdominal walls is used in open and laparoscopic cholecystectomy surgeries. The transducer should be placed at the lower margin of the rib cage at level of axillary line between the xiphoid process and anterosuperior iliac spine. The needle under ultrasound guidance is inserted until it is positioned between anterior edge of the transverse abdominis and the posterior rectus sheath, thus blocking T6-9 dermatomes.
  2. *Lateral approach* for lateral abdominal wall laparoscopic surgeries, open appendicectomy, ventral hernia repair, etc., the transducer is placed in mid axillary line between subcostal bony prominence and iliac crest. The needle should be located in plane between transverse abdominis and internal oblique muscles, thus blocking T10-12 dermatomes.
  3. *Posterior approach* for nephrectomies, renal transplant, anterolateral compartment of abdominal wall, etc., the transducer is placed in midaxillary line and moved posteriorly till the muscle compartment ends. The local anesthetic is deposited in plane between transverse abdominis and internal oblique, but at posterior end limit, it blocks T9-12 dermatomes.

SIDE EFFECT[4,14]

Discomfort at injection site.

COMPLICATIONS[2,4,13]

- Infection
- Bleeding/hematoma
- Local anesthetic toxicity
- Vascular puncture
- Intravascular toxicity
- Needle-induced paresthesia

SUMMARY

- TAP blocks do not provide anesthesia for surgery as it has no effect on visceral anesthesia or analgesia, so used as adjunctive for analgesia only.
- TAP blocks are a fascial plane technique and deliver local anesthesia around small abdominal wall nerves and anesthetize them.

REFERENCES

1. Mahmoud S, Miraflor E, Martin D, Mantuani D, Luftig J, Nagdev AD. Ultrasound-guided transverse abdominis plane block for ED appendicitis pain control. Am J Emerg Med. 2019;37(4):740-3.
2. El-Dawlatly AA, Turkistani A, Kettner SC, Machata AM, Delvi MB, Thallaj A, et al. Ultrasound-guided transversus abdominis plane block: description of a new technique and comparison with conventional systemic analgesia during laparoscopic cholecystectomy. Br J Anaesth. 2009;102(6):763-7.
3. Tran DQ, Bravo D, Leurcharusmee P, Neal JM. Transversus Abdominis Plane Block: Reply. Anesthesiology. 2020 Jun;132(6):1599. doi: 10.1097/ALN.0000000000003243. PMID: 32167980.
4. Mavarez AC, Hendrix JM, Ahmed AA. Transabdominal Plane Block. [Updated 2023 Nov 13]. In: StatPearls [Internet]. Treasure Island (FL): StatPearls Publishing; 2025 Jan-. Available from: https://www.ncbi.nlm.nih.gov/books/NBK560527/

5. O'Donnell BD, McDonnell JG, McShane AJ. The transversus abdominis plane (TAP) block in open retropubic prostatectomy. Reg Anesth Pain Med. 2006;31(1):91. [Erratum in: Reg Anesth Pain Med. 2006;31(3):286].
6. Bhowmick LK, Mahabubuzzaman M, Islam MS, Kabir MH. Study of analgesic effect of magnesium sulphate with bupivacaine in ultrasonogram guided transversus abdominis plane block for post-operative analgesia in lower uterine cesarean section. Commun Med J. 2021;10(1):9-17.
7. Aggarwal AK, Ottestad E, Pfaff KE, Huai-Yu Li A, Xu L, Derby R, et al. Review of ultrasound-guided procedures in the management of chronic pain. Anesthesiol Clin. 2023;41(2):395-470.
8. Elsharydah A, De La Cruz R, Horani SM, Xiao CY. Utilization of truncal fascial plane nerve blocks for chronic pain management: a narrative review. Curr Pain Headache Rep. 2023;27(6):149-55.
9. Tsai HC, Yoshida T, Chuang TY, Yang SF, Chang CC, Yao HY, et al. Transversus abdominis plane block: an updated review of anatomy and techniques. Biomed Res Int. 2017;2017:8284363.
10. Ripollés J, Mezquita SM, Abad A, Calvo J. Analgesic efficacy of the ultrasound-guided blockade of the transversus abdominis plane-a systematic review. Rev Bras Anestesiol. 2015;65:255-80.
11. Abdallah FW, Chan VW, Brull R. Transversus abdominis plane block: a systematic review. Reg Anesth Pain Med. 2012;37(2):193-209.
12. Nagata J, Watanabe J, Nagata M, Sawatsubashi Y, Akiyama M, Tajima T, et al. Transperitoneal rectus sheath block and transversus abdominis plane block for laparoscopic inguinal hernia repair: a novel approach. Asian J Endosc Surg. 2017;10(3):336-8.
13. Sharma D, Meena S, Anand G. Randomized single blind trial to compare the short term post-operative outcome and cost analysis of laparoscopic versus ultrasound guided transversus abdominis plane block in patients undergoing bariatric surgery. Surg Endosc. 2023;37(9):7136-43.
14. Prabhakar P, Ganapathi HP, Suresh V, Farias A, Manoharan M. Surgeon administered transversus abdominis plane block: anatomic principles and technique. J Robot Surg. 2023;17(4):1193-205.

CHAPTER 10

Greater Occipital Nerve Block

INTRODUCTION

The dysfunction of greater occipital nerve upper neck and occipital region and on its dysfunction results in severe headaches such as occipital neuralgia, migraine, cluster headache, and cervicogenic headache. The greater occipital nerve block (GONB) under ultrasound guidance can be beneficial in these headaches.[1-3]

IMPORTANT ANATOMICAL CONSIDERATIONS

The greater occipital nerve is one of the three nerves and largest nerve arising from C2-C3 spinal nerves innervating posterior scalp, other two being lesser occipital and third occipital nerve.[4] The GON share common sensory innervation with trigeminal nucleus caudalis creating a common nociceptive continuum between trigeminal and cervical fiber, thus GONB is helpful in many primary and secondary headaches.[5-8]

INDICATIONS[9-11]

- Occipital neuralgia
- Migraine
- Cluster headache
- Postdural puncture headache
- Cervicogenic headache

CONTRAINDICATIONS[12,13]

- *Absolute:*
  - Local anesthetic allergy
  - Patient refusal
  - Open skull defect
  - Infection at the local paraspinal site
  - Lack of skilled assistance
  - Lack of resuscitation equipment
- *Relative:*
  - Deranged coagulation
  - Systemic infection
  - Arnold-Chiari malformation

EQUIPMENT[14]

Healthcare professionals performing infraclavicular block should be equipped with the following items:

- Standard physiological monitors [electrocardiogram (ECG), BP apparatus, and pulse oximeter]
- Resuscitation equipment
- Ultrasound machine with a linear transducer (6–12 MHz)
- Sterile gloves, drapes, and ultrasonography (USG) probe covers
- Skin antiseptics, e.g., betadine, alcohol, and chlorhexidine
- Local anesthetic, i.e., 2% lidocaine
- Mild sedative agents, i.e., 1–2 mg of midazolam
- Regional block local anesthesia 20–30 mL (0.25% bupivacaine/2% lidocaine)
- 25-gauge nerve block needle
- A 5-mL syringe with a 25-gauge needle with local anesthetic agent for skin infiltration
- One 5-mL syringe with local anesthetic
- Methyl prednisolone (40 mg/mL)/dexamethasone (2 mg/mL)
- Marking pen

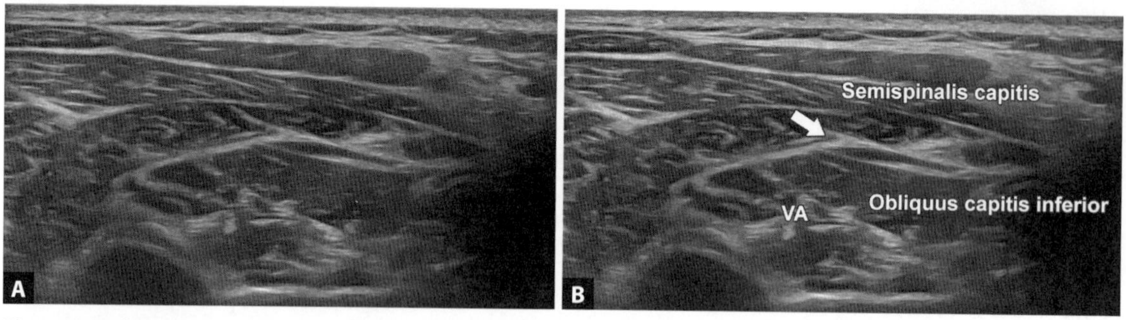

Figs. 1A and B: Sonographic anatomy form superficial to deep plane to localize greater occipital nerve in occipital region seen as hypoechoic oval structure (white thick arrow), overlying it is semispinalis capitis muscle and underlying is obliquus capitis inferior muscle, the vertebral artery (VA) is also seen.

PERSONNEL

An anesthesiologist with experience of regional anesthesia will require an additional person who will assist and monitor the vitals of the patient and will administer the emergency drugs if needed.[1,11]

ULTRASONOGRAPHY-GUIDED GREATER OCCIPITAL NERVE BLOCK TECHNIQUE[4,10,11]

- The provider must perform the process of informed consent.
- Gain intravenous access, apply standard monitors, and perform standard safety checklist.
- *Patient positioning:* The patient can be positioned in the supine position and with neck extended. The clinician performing the block and ultrasound machine should be placed ergonomically.
- Mild sedation with 1–2 mg of midazolam may be provided though many patients do not need it.
- Skin antiseptic is applied to the skin, then sterile conduction gel is applied to the ultrasound transducer, and use of sterile probe cover is recommended.
- *Transducer positioning and technique:*[10-12] The linear high-frequency transducer is placed in transverse orientation inferior to external occipital protuberance. The probe is then moved inferior till bifid tubercles of C2 spinous process is visualized. Then transducer is moved laterally tuned in oblique orientation till it is parallel to obliquus capitis inferior muscle and cephalad is semispinalis capitis muscle. The greater occipital nerve is in the fascial plane in between the two muscles seen as hypoechoic structure (**Figs. 1A and B**). After anesthetizing the skin, the needle is advanced under in plane and hydrodissection techniques to this location carefully by frequent aspirations. 3–5 mL of local anesthetic is injected slowly and should be visualized as fascial plane distension and spread around the nerve.

SIDE EFFECTS[13-15]

- Infection
- Nerve injury
- Allergic reaction
- Local anesthetic toxicity

COMPLICATIONS[16]

- Nerve damage
- Vessel puncture
- Subarachnoid space injection

SUMMARY

Ultrasound-guided GONB is a useful technique for variety of headache management and has proven to be minimally invasive and potentially effective.

REFERENCES

1. Lim HB, Hunt K. Anesthetic management for surgical placement of greater occipital nerve stimulators in the treatment of primary headache disorders. J Neurosurg Anesthesiol. 2007;19(2): 120-4.
2. Bogduk N. The clinical anatomy of the cervical dorsal rami. Spine (Phila Pa 1976). 1982;7(4): 319-30.
3. Urits I, Schwartz RH, Patel P, Zeien J, Connor D, Hasoon J, et al. A review of the recent findings in minimally invasive treatment options for the management of occipital neuralgia. Neurol Ther. 2020;9:229-41.
4. Harbell MW, Bolton PB, Koyyalamudi V, Seamans DP, Langley NR. Evaluating the anatomic spread of selective nerve scalp blocks using methylene blue: a cadaveric analysis. J Neurosurg Anesthesiol. 2023;35(2):248-52.
5. Fernandes L, Randall M MD FRCP, Idrovo L DMed FRCP. Peripheral nerve blocks for headache disorders. Pract Neurol. 2020: practneurol-2020-002612.
6. Levin M. Nerve blocks in the treatment of headache. Neurotherapeutics. 2010;7(2):197-203.
7. Inan N, Ceyhan A, Inan L, Kavaklioglu O, Alptekin A, Unal N. C2/C3 nerve blocks and greater occipital nerve block in cervicogenic headache treatment. Funct Neurol. 2001;16(3):239-43.
8. Blumenfeld A, Ashkenazi A, Napchan U, Bender SD, Klein BC, Berliner R, et al. Expert consensus recommendations for the performance of peripheral nerve blocks for headaches—a narrative review. Headache. 2013;53(3):437-46.
9. Tepper SJ, Stillman MJ. Cluster headache: potential options for medically refractory patients (when all else fails). Headache. 2013;53(7):1183-90.
10. Láinez MJ, Guillamón E. Cluster headache and other TACs: Pathophysiology and neurostimulation options. Headache. 2017;57(2): 327-35.
11. Miller S, Matharu M. Non-invasive Neuromodulation in primary headaches. Curr Pain Headache Rep. 2017;21(3):14.
12. Pincherle A, Bolyn S. Cerebellar syndrome after occipital nerve block: a case report. Cephalalgia. 2020;40(10):1123-6.
13. Austin M, Hinson MR. Occipital Nerve Block. In: StatPearls. Treasure Island (FL): StatPearls Publishing; 2025.
14. Brandt RB, Doesborg PGG, Meilof R, de Coo IF, Bartels E, Ferrari MD, et al. Repeated greater occipital nerve injections with corticosteroids in medically intractable chronic cluster headache: a retrospective study. Neurol Sci. 2022; 43(2):1267-72.
15. Chu XL, Song XZ, Li YR, Wu ZR, Li Q, Li QW, et al. An ultrasound-guided percutaneous electrical nerve stimulation regimen devised using finite element modeling promotes functional recovery after median nerve transection. Neural Regen Res. 2023;18(3):683-8.
16. Kumar P, Singh A, Sharma J, Parshad S, Johar S, Kaur K. Assessment of ultrasound guided erector spinae plane block for early post-operative analgesia for modified radical mastectomy: a prospective, randomized, controlled study. Med Gas Res. 2024;14(4):201-5.

CHAPTER 11

Superior Laryngeal Nerve Block

INTRODUCTION

The superior laryngeal nerve block (SLNB), a regional anesthesia technique, can effectively abolish the glottic closer reflex and the blunt sensations of the structure above the cords, thus aiding in awake tracheal intubation. The awake intubation of trachea is aimed at placing a tracheal tube in a wake spontaneously breathing patient with goal of achieving airway maintenance.[1-3]

IMPORTANT ANATOMICAL CONSIDERATIONS

The superior laryngeal nerve supplies sensation to the laryngeal structures above the vocal cords and is located in the inferior aspect of the greater cornu of the hyoid bone where it is divided into internal and external branches.[1,4]

INDICATIONS[5,6]

- Awake intubation
- Neurogenic cough
- Hypersensitive larynx resulting in dysphonia
- Inducible laryngeal obstruction
- Isolated globus pharyngeus

CONTRAINDICATIONS[6,7]

- *Absolute:*
  - Local anesthetic allergy
  - Patient refusal
  - Infection at the local paraspinal site
  - Lack of skilled assistance
  - Lack of resuscitation equipment
- *Relative:*
  - Deranged coagulation
  - Systemic infection
  - Laryngeal edema and pharyngitis
  - Severe respiratory disease
  - Recent use of sedatives

EQUIPMENT[8]

Healthcare professionals performing infraclavicular block should be equipped with the following items:

- Standard physiological monitors [electrocardiogram (ECG), BP apparatus, and pulse oximeter]
- Resuscitation equipment
- Ultrasound machine with a linear transducer (6– 12 MHz)
- Sterile gloves, drapes, and ultrasonography (USG) probe covers
- Skin antiseptics, e.g., betadine, alcohol, and chlorhexidine
- Local anesthetic, i.e., 2% lidocaine
- Mild sedative agents, i.e., 1–2 mg of midazolam
- Regional block local anesthesia 20–30 mL (0.25% bupivacaine/2% lidocaine)
- 23–25-gauge nerve block needle
- A 3-mL syringe with a 25-gauge needle with local anesthetic agent for skin infiltration
- One 5-mL syringe with local anesthetic
- Cotton swab soaked in 4% lignocaine solution
- Marking pen

PERSONNEL

An anesthesiologist with experience of regional anesthesia will require an additional person who will assist and monitor the vitals of the patient and will administer the emergency drugs if needed.[1,9]

ULTRASONOGRAPHY-GUIDED SUPERIOR LARYNGEAL NERVE BLOCK TECHNIQUE[9–11]

- The provider must perform the process of informed consent.
- Gain intravenous access, apply standard monitors, and perform standard safety checklist.
- *Patient positioning*: The patient can be positioned in the supine position and with neck extended. The clinician performing the block and ultrasound machine should be placed ergonomically.
- Mild sedation with 1–2 mg of midazolam may be provided though many patients do not need it.
- Skin antiseptic is applied to the skin, then sterile conduction gel is applied to the ultrasound transducer, and use of sterile probe cover is recommended.
- To minimize the secretions in the airway, 0.2 mg of glycopyrrolate is administered.

Transducer positioning and technique:[9,11,12] The linear ultrasound transducer is placed in longitudinal orientation in submandibular and the greater horn of hyoid bone and thyroid cartilage are identified which appear as hyperechoic on sonography **(Figs. 1A and B)**. The thyrohyoid muscle and thyrohyoid membrane are identified between these structures and in-between them lies the internal branch of superior laryngeal nerve seen as hypoechoic structure. The block is performed with 25-gauge needle tips traversed through anesthetized skin by in plane technique by 5 mL syringe 2% lidocaine, 1.5 mL on each side.

SIDE EFFECTS[13,14]

- Dysphagia
- Dyspnea
- Aspiration
- Infection
- Nerve injury
- Allergic reaction
- Local anesthetic toxicity

COMPLICATIONS[13,14]

- Laryngeal anesthesia
- Nerve damage
- Vessel puncture
- Bleeding/hematoma
- Failed block

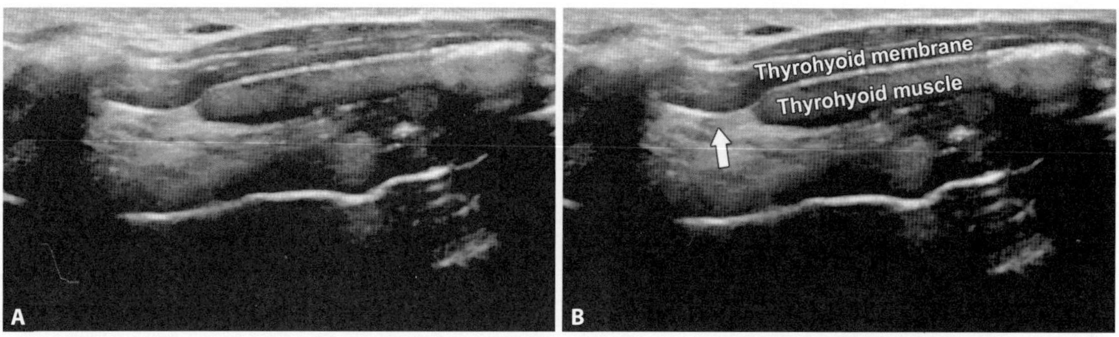

Figs. 1A and B: Sonographic anatomy of superior laryngeal nerve block with arrow showing superior laryngeal nerve and labeled anatomic structures thyrohyoid membrane and thyrohyoid muscle.

SUMMARY

- The use of ultrasound-guided block of superior laryngeal nerve is an important tool in the management of difficult airways.
- It is used in various surgery, treating neurogenic cough, managing laryngeal pain and as adjunct to topical anesthesia for various upper airway procedures.

REFERENCES

1. Hua Y, Huang Q, Chen G, Zhu T. Comparison of modified anterior and traditional posterior accesses for ultrasound-guided superior laryngeal nerve block in awake endotracheal intubation: study protocol for a randomised non-inferiority clinical trial. BMJ Open. 2023;13:e068779.
2. Liao YC, Wu WC, Hsieh MH, Chang CC, Tsai HC. Ultrasound-guided superior laryngeal nerve block assists in anesthesia for bronchoscopic surgical procedure: A case report of anesthesia for rigid bronchoscopy. Medicine (Baltimore). 2020;99(27)e20916.
3. Simmons ST, Schleich AR. Airway regional anesthesia for awake fiberoptic intubation. Reg Anesth Pain Med. 2002;27(2):180-92.
4. Gotta AW, Sullivan CA. Anaesthesia of the upper airway using topical anaesthetic and superior laryngeal nerve block. Br J Anaesth. 1981;53(10):1055-8.
5. Lan CH, Cheng WC, Yang YL. A new method for ultrasound-guided superior laryngeal nerve block. Tzu Chi Med J. 2013;25(3):161-3.
6. Gray AJ, Hoffman MR, Yang ZM, Vandiver B, Purvis J, Morgan JP, et al. Indications and Short-Term Outcomes for In-Office Therapeutic Superior Laryngeal Nerve Block. Ann Otol Rhinol Laryngol. 2024;133(2):174-80.
7. Ahmad I, El-Boghdadly K, Bhagrath R, Hodzovic I, McNarry AF, Mir F, et al. Difficult Airway Society guidelines for awake tracheal intubation (ATI) in adults. Anaesthesia. 2020;75(4):509-28.
8. Kojima Y, Sugimura M. Superior Laryngeal Nerve Block for Intubation in Patients With COVID-19. Anesth Prog. 2021;68(1):50-1.
9. Ambi US, Arjun BK, Masur S, Endigeri A, Hosalli V, Hulakund SY. Comparison of ultrasound and anatomical landmark-guided technique for superior laryngeal nerve block to aid awake fibre-optic intubation: A prospective randomised clinical study. Indian J Anaesth. 2017;61(6):463-8.
10. Furlan JC. Anatomical study applied to anesthetic block technique of the superior laryngeal nerve. Acta Anaesth Scand. 2002;46(2):199-202.
11. Zhipeng L, Meiyi H, Meirong W, Qunmeng J, Zhenhua J, Yuezhen H, et al. Ultrasound-guided internal branch of superior laryngeal nerve block on postoperative sore throat: a randomized controlled trial. PLoS One. 2020;15(11):e0241834.
12. Magadum NB, Nileshwar A, Vijayakumara. Comparison of landmark-guided and ultrasound-guided technique for superior laryngeal nerve block to aid fibreoptic intubation—An observational study. J Anaesthesiol Clin Pharmacol. 2023;39(2):226-31.
13. Dhillon VK. Longitudinal Follow-up of Superior Laryngeal Nerve Block for Chronic Neurogenic Cough. OTO Open. 2021;5(1):2473974X21994468.
14. Malta SM, Bilotta F, Nozari A. Is it Safe to Use Ultrasound-Guided Superior Laryngeal Nerve Block for the Prevention of Postoperative Sore Throat After Double Lumen Endotracheal Intubation? Anesth Analg. 2024;138(1):e1-2.

SECTION 4

Lower Limb Blocks

CHAPTER 12

Femoral Nerve Block

INTRODUCTION

The peripheral nerve blocks inhibit the impulse propagation in nerve terminalis thus inhibits its perception in the cerebral cortex. The femoral nerve block under ultrasound guidance causes the femoral nerve blockade, allowing the practitioner to visualize and monitor the needle placement and desirable deposition of local anesthetic.[1-4] This block is preferred as it is relatively superficial, easily identified structures sonographically and complications are low.[5]

IMPORTANT ANATOMICAL CONSIDERATIONS

The femoral nerve is derived from the anterior rami of the nerve roots from L2-L4, and it emerges below lateral border of psoas muscle and enters the anterior of thigh underneath the inguinal ligament dividing into two divisions (anterior and posterior).[3]

INDICATIONS[2]

- Surgeries of knee
- Analgesia in femoral neck fracture, femur fracture, and patellar injuries
- Multimodal pain management

CONTRAINDICATIONS[4,6]

- *Absolute:*
  - Local anesthetic allergy
  - Patient refusal
  - Infection at the local site
  - Lack of skilled assistance
  - Lack of resuscitation equipment
- *Relative:*
  - Deranged coagulation
  - Systemic infection
  - Preexisting nerve damage

EQUIPMENT[2,3]

Healthcare professionals performing infraclavicular block should be equipped with the following items:

- Standard physiological monitors [electrocardiogram (ECG), BP apparatus, and pulse oximeter]
- Resuscitation equipment
- Ultrasound machine with a high-frequency linear transducer (8–15 MHz)
- Sterile gloves, drapes, and ultrasonography (USG) probe covers
- Skin antiseptics, e.g., betadine, alcohol, and chlorhexidine
- Local anesthetic, i.e., 2% lidocaine
- Mild sedative agents, i.e., 1–2 mg of midazolam
- Regional block local anesthesia (0.25% bupivacaine, rest 0.2% ropivacaine/2% lidocaine for postoperative analgesia)
- Short bevel insulated, stimulating block needle 50–100 mm (22-gauge for single injection and 18 gauge for continuous catheter), insulated, stimulating needle
- A 3-mL syringe with a 25-gauge needle with local anesthetic agent for skin infiltration
- One 20-mL syringe with local anesthetic
- Marking pen

PERSONNEL

The femoral nerve block requires two persons, one to control the ultrasound probe and needle and the other person will manage the syringe with local anesthetic. Additional person will also monitor the vitals of the patient and will administer the emergency drugs if needed [4,6]

ULTRASONOGRAPHY-GUIDED FEMORAL NERVE BLOCK TECHNIQUE [7,8]

- The provider must perform the process of informed consent.
- Gain intravenous access, apply standard monitors, and perform standard safety checklist[8]
- *Patient positioning:* The patient can be positioned in supine position with the limb in contention is straight, in slight abduction, and in slight external rotation.[4]
- Mild sedation with 1–2 mg of midazolam may be provided though many patients do not need it.[3]
- Skin antiseptic is applied to the skin, then sterile conduction gel is applied to the ultrasound transducer, and use of sterile probe cover is recommended.[1,2] The block can be performed awake or under sedation.[2]
- *Transducer positioning and technique:*[2,3] The high-frequency linear transducer is placed at the inguinal crease transversely over the inguinal crease and the common femoral artery and femoral vein is localized. The femoral nerve is seen as hyperechoic structure lateral to femoral vessels. The femoral nerve lies beneath skin, subcutaneous tissue, fascia lata, and fascia iliaca, which covers iliopsoas muscle, sartorius muscle belly is seen anterolaterally. The femoral artery and vein are seen medially encased in femoral sheath, and the femoral nerve is seen outside of the femoral sheath **(Figs. 1A and B)**.[4,6,9] On identification of the various structures, the short bevel bloc needle is advanced in in-plane technique with needle tip advanced the fascia iliaca toward the femoral nerve. The local anesthetic is injected with frequent negative aspirates to avoid intravascular injections, and the quantity of the injection is monitored through the ultrasound screen. The intraneural injection is also avoided, which is seen as neural expansion on injecting.[10,11]

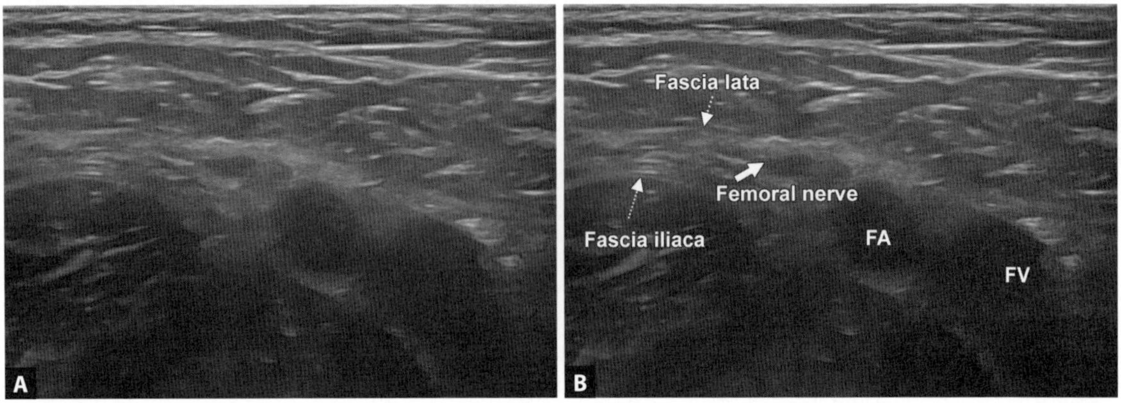

Figs. 1A and B: Sonographic anatomy of femoral nerve plane from superficial to deep and arrow indicating sciatic nerve and the local anesthetic spread should be around the nerve, fascia lata, and fascia Iliaca are also seen marked in dotted arrows.

SIDE EFFECTS[10,12]

- Discomfort at injection site
- Difficulty with mobility, patients should not be ambulated without assistance after the block

COMPLICATIONS[2,10,12]

- Infection
- Bleeding/hematoma
- Local anesthetic toxicity
- Vascular puncture
- Intravascular toxicity
- Needle-induced paresthesia
- Permanent nerve injury

SUMMARY[13]

- The femoral nerve block blocks motor as well as sensory nerves.
- It can be used as one of the useful adjuncts for postoperative analgesia.
- The use of ultrasound adds to the precision, faster block, and reduction in the requirement of the dose.

REFERENCES

1. Atchabahian A, Leunen I, Vandepitte C, Lopez AM. Ultrasound-Guided Femoral Nerve Block. In: Hadzic A (Ed). Hadzic's Textbook of Regional Anesthesia and Acute Pain Management, 2nd edition. McGraw-Hill Education; 2017.
2. Sykes, Zahra, and Aimee Pak. "Femoral nerve block." (2019).
3. Pepall T. Ultrasound Guided Femoral Nerve Block. Anaesthesia. Tutorial of the Week 284. 15th April 2013.
4. Kasibhatla RD, Russon K. Femoral nerve blocks. J Perioper Pract. 2009;19(2):65-9.
5. Wang AZ, Gu L, Zhou QH, Ni WZ, Jiang W. Ultrasound-guided continuous femoral nerve block for analgesia after total knee arthroplasty: catheter perpendicular to the nerve versus catheter parallel to the nerve. Reg Anesth Pain Med. 2010;35(2):127-31.
6. Sandby-Thomas M, Sullivan G, Hall JE. A national survey into the peri-operative anaesthetic management of patients presenting for surgical correction of a fractured neck of femur. Anaesthesia. 2008;63(3):250-8.
7. Becker DE, Reed KL. Local anesthetics: review of pharmacological considerations. Anesth Prog. 2012 Summer;59(2):90-101; quiz 102-3.
8. Neal JM, Woodward CM, Harrison TK. The American Society of Regional Anesthesia and Pain Medicine Checklist for Managing Local Anesthetic Systemic Toxicity: 2017 Version. Reg Anesth Pain Med. 2018;43(2):150-3.
9. Behera SK, Gunupuru B, Sahu L, Das S. Peripheral Nerve Stimulator Versus Ultrasound-Guided Femoral Nerve Block for Knee Arthroscopy Procedures: A Randomized Controlled Trial. Cureus. 2022;14(11):e32043.
10. Nagel EM, Gantioque R, Taira T. Utilizing Ultrasound-Guided Femoral Nerve Blocks and Fascia Iliaca Compartment Blocks for Proximal Femur Fractures in the Emergency Department. Adv Emerg Nurs J. 2019;41(2):135-44.
11. Mariano ER, Loland VJ, Sandhu NS, Bellars RH, Bishop ML, Afra R, et al. Ultrasound guidance versus electrical stimulation for femoral perineural catheter insertion. J Ultrasound Med. 2009;28(11):1453-60.
12. Chan EY, Fransen M, Parker DA, Assam PN, Chua N. Femoral nerve blocks for acute postoperative pain after knee replacement surgery. Cochrane Database Syst Rev. 2014;2014(5):CD009941.
13. Munirama S, McLeod G. Ultrasound-guided femoral and sciatic nerve blocks. Continuing Educ Anaesth Crit Care Pain. 2013;13(4):136-40.

CHAPTER 13

Sciatic Nerve Block

INTRODUCTION

The sciatic nerve block provides sensory as well as motor innervation of the lower limb and is commonly used for its anesthesia or analgesia. The ultrasound guidance for regional anesthetic blockade of the sciatic nerve has now become a standard practice.[1,2]

IMPORTANT ANATOMICAL CONSIDERATIONS

The sacral plexus formed from the anterior rami of L4-L5 of the lumbosacral trunk and sciatic nerve is the major branch of the sacral plexus, which exits the pelvis through the greater sciatic foramen below piriformis muscle. It then descends inferolateral and is located under gluteus maximus between greater trochanter and ischial tuberosity. The sciatic nerve then enters the posterior thigh anterior to long head of biceps femoris and as it approaches the apex of popliteal fossa it divides into the tibial nerve and the common peroneal nerve.[1,3,4]

INDICATIONS[2,5]

- Ankle surgery
- Hindfoot surgery
- Midfoot surgery
- Below knee amputation
- Total knee replacement
- Acute and chronic pain management of lower limb

CONTRAINDICATIONS[2,6]

- *Absolute:*
  - Local anesthetic allergy
  - Patient refusal
  - Infection at the local site
  - Lack of skilled assistance
  - Lack of resuscitation equipment
- *Relative:*
  - Deranged coagulation
  - Systemic infection
  - Documented neurological disease or deficit

EQUIPMENT[2,3,7]

Healthcare professionals performing infraclavicular block should be equipped with the following items:

- Standard physiological monitors [electrocardiogram (ECG), BP apparatus, and pulse oximeter]
- Resuscitation equipment
- Ultrasound machine with a curvilinear transducer (2–5 MHz)
- Sterile gloves, drapes, and ultrasonography (USG) probe covers
- Skin antiseptics, e.g., betadine, alcohol, and chlorhexidine
- Local anesthetic, i.e., 2% lidocaine
- Mild sedative agents, i.e., 1–2 mg of midazolam
- Regional block local anesthesia (0.25% bupivacaine, rest are/0.2% ropivacaine/2% lidocaine for postoperative analgesia)
- Short bevel insulated, stimulating block needle 50–100 mm (22-gauge for single injection and 18 gauge for continuous catheter), insulated, stimulating needle
- A 3-mL syringe with a 25-gauge needle with local anesthetic agent for skin infiltration

- One 20-mL syringe with local anesthetic
- Marking pen

PERSONNEL

The sciatic nerve block requires two persons, one to control the ultrasound probe and needle, other will manage the syringe with local anesthetic. He will also monitor the vitals of the patient and will administer the emergency drugs if needed.[2,3]

ULTRASONOGRAPHY-GUIDED SCIATIC NERVE BLOCK TECHNIQUE[7-9]

- The provider must perform the process of informed consent.
- Gain intravenous access, apply standard monitors, and perform standard safety check list.
- *Patient positioning:* The patient can be positioned in three positions:
  1. *Supine position:* Knee is kept straight with support under the lower leg; in this transducer, manipulations are easy.
  2. *Lateral:* As the side to be blocked is uppermost.
  3. Prone
- Mild sedation with 1–2 mg of midazolam may be provided though many patients do not need it.
- Skin antiseptic is applied to the skin, then sterile conduction gel is applied to the ultrasound transducer, and use of sterile probe cover is recommended. The block can be performed awake or under sedation.
- *Transducer positioning and technique:*[2,3,5,10-13] The curved transducer can be placed as per approach:
  - *Anterior approach:* With patients in supine position and transducer in transverse position on the proximal thigh around 8 cm distal to the inguinal crease to first visualize the femur, sliding medially to identify the adductor muscles, the sciatic nerve is located deep to adductor magnus and is posteromedial to the femur **(Figs. 1A and B)**.
  - *Subgluteal approach:* With the patient in lateral position and transducer placed in transverse plane sciatic nerve is visualized along a line between the greater trochanter and ischial tuberosity in the subgluteal fascial plane above the quadratus femoris.
  - *Popliteal approach:* With the patient positioned in supine and lateral position, first the popliteal artery is visualized in the crease of the knee and tibial nerve lying posterior to it followed by the probe proximally until the common peroneal

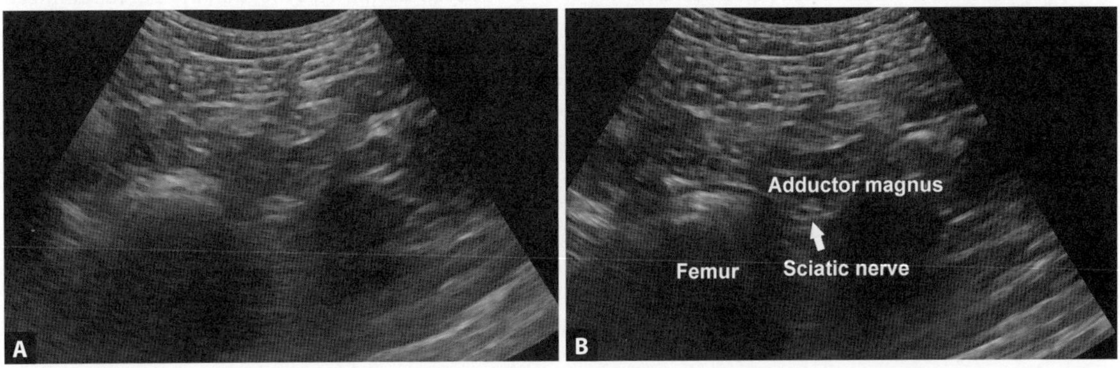

Figs. 1A and B: Sonographic anatomy of sciatic nerve plane from superficial to deep and white arrow indicating sciatic nerve and the local anesthetic spread should be around the nerve.

nerve joins to form sciatic nerve where the block is given.

The needle tip is inserted by in plane technique taking care not to traverse neurovascular bundles and 20 mL of local anesthetic is used in hydrodissection method with frequent negative aspirations to avoid intravascular injection.

SIDE EFFECTS[14]

- Discomfort at injection site
- Difficulty with mobility, the patient should not be ambulated without assistance after the block

COMPLICATIONS[2,14,15]

- Infection
- Bleeding/hematoma
- Local anesthetic toxicity
- Vascular puncture
- Intravascular toxicity
- Needle-induced paresthesia
- Permanent nerve injury

SUMMARY

- The sciatic nerve block blocks motor as well as sensory nerves providing anesthesia and analgesia to a wide range of lower limb procedures.
- The ultrasound guidance allows identification and localization of anatomical landmarks.
- The use of ultrasound adds to the precision, faster block, and reduction in the requirement of the dose.

REFERENCES

1. Rodziewicz TL, Stevens JB, Ajib FA, Tunnell DJ. Sciatic nerve block. In: StatPearls. Treasure Island (FL): StatPearls Publishing; 2023.
2. D'Souza RS, Hooten WM. Neurolytic Blocks. In: StatPearls. Treasure Island (FL): StatPearls Publishing; 2025.
3. Shevlin S, Johnston D, Turbitt L. The sciatic nerve block. BJA Educ. 2020;20(9):312-20.
4. Vloka JD, Hadzić A, April E, Thys DM. The division of the sciatic nerve in the popliteal fossa: anatomical implications for popliteal nerve blockade. Anesth Analg. 2001;92(1):215-7.
5. Mori T, Hagiwara Y. Ultrasound-Guided Popliteal Sciatic Nerve Block for an Ankle Laceration in a Pediatric Emergency Department. Pediatr Emerg Care. 2017;33(12):803-5.
6. Grape S, Kirkham KR, Baeriswyl M, Albrecht E. The analgesic efficacy of sciatic nerve block in addition to femoral nerve block in patients undergoing total knee arthroplasty: a systematic review and meta-analysis. Anaesthesia. 2016; 71(10):1198-209.
7. Gray AT, Collins AB, Schafhalter-Zoppoth I. Sciatic nerve block in a child: a sonographic approach. Anesth Analg. 2003;97(5):1300-2.
8. McCartney CJ, Brauner I, Chan VW. Ultrasound guidance for a lateral approach to the sciatic nerve in the popliteal fossa. Anaesthesia. 2004;59(10):1023-5.
9. Sinha A, Chan VW. Ultrasound imaging for popliteal sciatic nerve block. Reg Anesth Pain Med. 2004;29(2):130-4.
10. Johnston DF, Sondekoppam RV, Uppal V, Howard JL, Ganapathy S. Hybrid Blocks for Total Knee Arthroplasty: A Technical Description. Clin J Pain. 2018;34(3):222-30.
11. Wiederhold BD, Garmon EH, Peterson E, Stevens JB, O'Rourke MC. Nerve Block Anesthesia. In: StatPearls. Treasure Island (FL): StatPearls Publishing; 2025.
12. Zorrilla-Vaca A, Li J. The role of sciatic nerve block to complement femoral nerve block in total knee arthroplasty: a meta-analysis of randomized controlled trials. J Anesth. 2018;32(3):341-50.
13. Perlas A, Wong P, Abdallah F, Hazrati LN, Tse C, Chan V. Ultrasound-guided popliteal block through a common paraneural sheath versus conventional injection: a prospective, randomized, double-blind study. Reg Anesth Pain Med. 2013;38(3):218-25.
14. Nwawka OK, Meyer R, Miller TT. Ultrasound-Guided Subgluteal Sciatic Nerve Perineural Injection: Report on Safety and Efficacy at a Single Institution. J Ultrasound Med. 2017;36(11): 2319-24.
15. O'Donnell R, Dolan J. Anaesthesia and analgesia for knee joint arthroplasty. BJA Educ. 2018;18(1):8-15.

SECTION 5

Recent Advances

CHAPTER 14

Artificial Intelligence in Ultrasound-guided Regional Anesthesia

Artificial intelligence (AI) is a field of computer science which uses various algorithms and computational resources, enabling the machines to simulate human intelligence in its thought process and actions.[1] The utilization of AI and machine learning applications is rising exponentially in various medical discipline including anesthesiology.[1,2] This revolutionary technology is changing the traditional anesthesia practices of patient risk stratification, anesthesia delivery system, patient perioperative monitoring, individualized anesthesia, and image analysis by an automated process.[3]

The mechanical tasks such as intubation, ventilation, and nerve blocks are being carried out by AI-trained robots.[4] The tasks such as intubation, nerve block, and endoscope placement are mainly done by trained physicians, and precision with which the procedure is being carried out depends on expertise. So, these automated robotic models increase the spectrum of users and also increase the accuracy of procedure being done.[5,6]

Regional blocks are one of the most common and evolving anesthesia techniques in present times, and for their success, good operative skills are required as safety and efficiency are required.[1,7]

As the identification region of nerve block region is of utmost importance, especially for operators who are not much skilled in ultrasound. The amalgamation of AI can overcome the limitation of prolonged experience, training, human fatigue, and sometimes failure to identify correct anatomical structure.[8]

Artificial intelligence can prove to be pivotal which can construct datasets and trained models of ultrasonographic images to explore a method that will identify the nerve block region.[9] In one of the AI subsets called machine learning, the computer is trained from data and algorithms, patterns are identified, and decision making is performed. In other subsets of AI called deep learning using convolutional neural network as human brain enabling these AI models involve in recognizing and processing images.[3,4]

Artificial intelligence can be used to augment the performance of operator performing the ultrasonography (USG)-guided nerve blocks from identifying needle tip to injecting local anesthetic and even identifying complications.[10]

Artificial intelligence has the potential to change the landscapes of image-guided regional anesthesia practice, but at present, certain limitations are there such as insufficient patient data, mannequin-based training models, lack of standardization, and ethical and legal concerns which need to be addressed to make it more robust.

REFERENCES

1. Bowness J, Varsou O, Turbitt L, Burkett-St Laurent D. Identifying anatomical structures on ultrasound: assistive artificial intelligence in ultrasound-guided regional anesthesia. Clin Anat. 2021;34(5):802-9.
2. Swain BP, Nag DS, Anand R, Kumar H, Ganguly PK, Singh N. Current evidence on artificial intelligence in regional anesthesia. World J Clin Cases. 2024;12(33):6613-9.

3. Hetherington J, Lessoway V, Gunka V, Abolmaesumi P, Rohling R. SLIDE: automatic spine level identification system using a deep convolutional neural network. Int J Comput Assist Radiol Surg. 2017;12(7):1189-98.
4. Balavenkatasubramanian J, Kumar S, Sanjayan RD. Artificial intelligence in regional anaesthesia. Indian J Anaesth. 2024;68(1):100-4.
5. Huang C, Zhou Y, Tan W, Qiu Z, Zhou H, Song Y, et al. Applying deep learning in recognizing the femoral nerve block region on ultrasound images. Ann Transl Med. 2019;7(18):453.
6. Smistad E, Iversen DH, Leidig L, Lervik Bakeng JB, Johansen KF, Lindseth F. Automatic segmentation and probe guidance for real-time assistance of ultrasound-guided femoral nerve blocks. Ultrasound Med Biol. 2017;43(1):218-26.
7. Zhao Y, Zheng S, Cai N, Zhang Q, Zhong H, Zhou Y, et al. Utility of artificial intelligence for real-time anatomical landmark identification in ultrasound-guided thoracic paravertebral block. J Digit Imaging. 2023;36(5):2051-9.
8. Ahiskalioglu A, Yayik AM, Karapinar YE, Tulgar S, Ciftci B. From ultrasound to artificial intelligence: a new era of the regional anesthesia. Minerva Anestesiol. 2022;88(7-8):640-2.
9. Erdem G, Ermiş Y, Özkan D. Peripheral nerve blocks and the use of artificial intelligence-assisted ultrasonography. J Clin Anesth. 2022;78:110597.
10. Gungor I, Gunaydin B, Oktar SO, M Buyukgebiz B, Bagcaz S, Ozdemir MG, et al. A real-time anatomy identification via tool based on artificial intelligence for ultrasound-guided peripheral nerve block procedures: an accuracy study. J Anesth. 2021;35(4):591-4.

Index

Page numbers followed by *f* refer to figure.